MYCOTOXINS - IMPACT AND MANAGEMENT STRATEGIES

Edited by **Patrick Berka Njobeh**
and **Francois Stepman**

Mycotoxins - Impact and Management Strategies
http://dx.doi.org/10.5772/intechopen.72353
Edited by Patrick Berka Njobeh and Francois Stepman

Contributors

Emmanuel Jnr Zuza, Amade Muitia, Ana Maria Mondjana, Rick L. Brandenburg, Manuel I.V Amane, Mateen Abbas, Titilayo Falade, Guillermo Téllez, Bruno Solis-Cruz, Daniel Hernandez-Patlan, Billy Hargis, Yasir Allah Ditta, Saima Mahad, Umar Bacha, Lindy Rose, Sheila Okoth, Belinda Janse Van Rensburg, Bradley Flett, Sefater Gbashi, Ifeoluwa Adekoya, Oluwafemi Ayodeji Adebo, Sarah De Saeger, Ntakadzeni Edwin Madala, Marthe De Boevre, Patrick Berka Njobeh, Mohamed Fathi Abdallah, Maarten Ameye, Kris Audenaert, Geert Haesaert

First published in London, United Kingdom, 2019 by IntechOpen
IntechOpen is the global imprint of INTECHOPEN LIMITED, registered in England and Wales, registration number: 11086078, The Shard, 25th floor, 32 London Bridge Street
London, SE19SG – United Kingdom
Printed in Croatia

British Library Cataloguing-in-Publication Data
A catalogue record for this book is available from the British Library

Additional hard and PDF copies can be obtained from orders@intechopen.com

Mycotoxins - Impact and Management Strategies, Edited by Patrick Berka Njobeh and Francois Stepman
p. cm.
Print ISBN 978-1-83881-846-3
Online ISBN 978-1-83881-847-0
eBook (PDF) ISBN 978-1-83881-848-7

For EU product safety concerns:
IN TECH d.o.o., Prolaz Marije Krucifikse Kozulić 3, 51000 Rijeka, Croatia,
info@intechopen.com or visit our website at intechopen.com.

Meet the editors

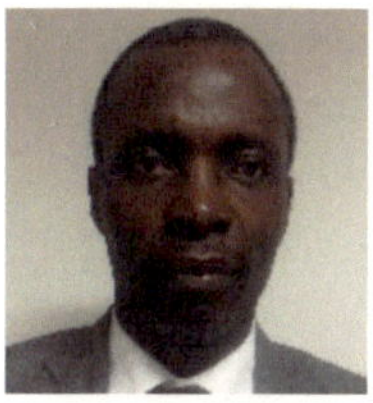

P.B. Njobeh is an associate professor and deputy head of the Department of Biotechnology and Food Technology and heads the Mycotoxin Unit of the University of Johannesburg (UJ), South Africa, with 21 postgraduates and postdoctoral fellows currently under his supervision. His research projects fall within the area of food safety, with an emphasis on mycotoxins and fungi. He has established research collaborations with various institutions nationally and internationally and is part of the MYTOX_SOUTH consortium, a partnership to improve food security and safety through mitigation of mycotoxins at a global level with Ghent University, Belgium, as leading partner. He is equally part of the iZindaba Zokudla, a multistakeholder program hosted at UJ aimed at creating opportunities for urban agriculture in a sustainable food system and engaging with the communities in Johannesburg and its environs on food-related issues. He also works as consultant/expert in the African Union Inter-Bureau on Animal Resources/African Union's projects, especially on food safety. He is a member of the Joint (FAO/WHO) Expert Committee on Food Additives, which is responsible for delivering scientific advice on the establishment of global food safety standards of Codex Alimentarius and others. Prof. Njobeh is a reviewer of more than 14 scientific journals, several funding applications for the National Research Foundation (NRF), Medical Research Council of South Africa and Research Foundation-Flanders, Belgium, an editorial board member of Mycotoxin Research, and an external examiner of theses and dissertations from other universities. He has more than 80 publications as book chapters and journal and conference papers. He is a reviewer for many journals and funding bodies, with a Google Scholar H-index of 16 and 889 citations, and a Scopus H-index of 13 with 560 citations. Prof. Njobeh is a C2 NRF-rated researcher and has attracted several research grants.

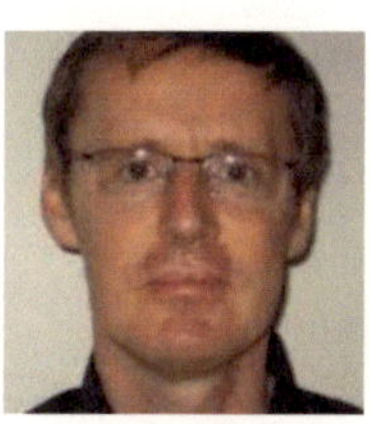

Francois Stepman is currently communications expert for the International Center for Agricultural Research in dry areas based in Cairo. Previously, he managed for a decade the communications of the Platform for African–European Partnership in Agricultural Research for Development (PAEPARD), which was funded by the European Commission. He has more than 20 years of experience in development cooperation, policy advisory research, and capacity building in Southern research institutes. He lived for approximately 10 years in Africa where he worked for the United Nations Development Programme in Mauritania, Medecins Sans Frontieres in South Sudan, and the Forum for Agricultural Research in Africa in Ghana. Over the past 10 years, he has been extensively blogging on agricultural issues in Africa.

The PAEPARD blog has an average of 25,000 visitors per month. In 2016, he convened at the European Commission a round table of experts on aflatoxin to endorse a policy brief on the contamination of food and feed with aflatoxin in Africa. He manages an online community of 10,800 members. This includes a subcommunity of 400 African and global mycotoxin experts, which assesses current research and development needs, available expertise, and opportunities for collaboration and the dissemination of reports and conferences related to food safety, in particular mycotoxin contamination.

Contents

Preface

Food and feed contamination by toxigenic fungi accompanied by the production of various mycotoxins is a serious concern worldwide because it seriously compromises health and the economy. This is more devastating in Africa due to climate change dynamics, food habits, poor perception, and the lack of public awareness and educational programs. Mycotoxins are the most important chronic dietary risk factor, ahead of synthetic contaminants, plant toxins, and pesticide residues, with aflatoxin B1 being the most potent naturally occurring carcinogen. As such, their presence in food and feed seriously compromises food and feed safety; thus, there is a need for their regulation and control.

Aflatoxin contamination of food and feed affects a wide variety of industries, including nutrition, agriculture, health, and trade. From a historical viewpoint, one can notice that over the past decades the interest of research, development cooperation agencies, or international health bodies to the problem of aflatoxin has received an unequal attention. Resurfacing in the international news in the 1990s, it faded away to once again reemerge due to increased attention from research funders and development actors to food safety issues and nutrition. In 2019 there is a crucial need for high-level discussion on food safety, including aflatoxin contamination. The Food and Agriculture Organization (FAO), World Health Organization (WHO), and World Trade Organization (WTO) organized an International Forum on Food Safety and Trade (23–24 April 2019. Geneva). This conference continued the discussions from the Addis Conference (12–13 February 2019. Addis Ababa) to address specifically the trade-related aspects and challenges of food safety.

However, collaboration between different actors is still challenging, not least because of the complexity of the contamination sources that occur at pre-harvest and post-harvest levels. Many initiatives and surveys have focused on how bad the situation is in some African countries and for some value chains. Less attention has been paid to understanding the reasons why it is so difficult to devise possible solutions that mitigate aflatoxin contamination to scale.

This book offers an opportunity for African scientists to present their current research results and demonstrates the great diversity of research topics. Section 1 covers the socioeconomic impact of mycotoxins, Section 2 looks into prevention and control of aflatoxins, and Section 3 discusses aflatoxicosis and control in poultry. The book contributes to the ambitious objectives of MYTOX-SOUTH, which was launched in 2017. This initiative intends to support the capacity of (mainly) African partners in their research on mycotoxin contamination and how it affects not only food safety but also food security. The well-structured multidisciplinary partnership of MYTOX-SOUTH deals with all known aspects of mycotoxins and toxigenic mold issues. The final goal is to contribute to formulating adequate strategies and solutions for different stakeholders who are affected by mycotoxin contamination.

It is hoped that the information contained in this book will be valuable to all and serve as an aid to students, researchers, and professionals involved in the field of mycotoxicology, as well as policy makers and regulatory bodies. Reports that try to model and forecast the impact of climate change on the African continent predict that many African regions will undergo periods of drought. For instance, East Africa will experience a hotter but also a more humid climate. This will exacerbate the situation in Africa, where the occurrence of aflatoxin is already more persistent than anywhere else across the globe.

Hence it is important to give more visibility to recent research on mycotoxins from an African perspective. The book is also an answer to the 2018 recommendations of the Joint FAO/WHO Expert Committee on Food Additives (JECFA). JEFCA recommended that efforts to reduce aflatoxin exposure using valid intervention strategies continue, including the development of effective, sustainable, and universally applicable pre-harvest prevention strategies. Rice, wheat, and sorghum need to be considered in future risk management activities for aflatoxins. JEFCA recommended further research and efforts to alleviate stunting, taking aflatoxin exposure into consideration as a possible contributing factor. It recommended that if additional epidemiological studies are conducted, they should be prospective studies that are performed in high-exposure areas (e.g., in Africa). It advises on the development of surveillance programs for regions for which little information on the occurrence of aflatoxins currently exists, carefully considering the impact of these programs on food security. I would like to sincerely thank my colleague Mr. Francois Stepman for his valuable contribution as co-editor and also Prof. Gabriel Adegoke of the University of Ibadan, Prof. Hussaini Makun of the Federal University of Technology Minna, Nigeria, and lastly Dr. Fru Felix of the University of Johannesburg for reviewing some of the chapters published herein. Finally, my profound gratitude goes to all authors who contributed to the book.

Patrick Berka Njobeh
Department of Biotechnology and Food Technology
Faculty of Science
University of Johannesburg, South Africa

Francois Stepman
The European Alliance on Agricultural Knowledge for Development/KEYSTEP bvba
Paris, France

Section 1

Socio-economic Impact of Mycotoxins

Chapter 1

The Socio-Economic Impact of Mycotoxin Contamination in Africa

Sefater Gbashi, Ntakadzeni Edwin Madala, Sarah De Saeger, Marthe De Boevre, Ifeoluwa Adekoya, Oluwafemi Ayodeji Adebo and Patrick Berka Njobeh

Additional information is available at the end of the chapter

http://dx.doi.org/10.5772/intechopen.79328

Abstract

The proliferated contamination of agricultural commodities by mycotoxins and their attendant toxic effects on humans and animals which consume such commodities constitutes a major concern to food safety and security. These highly toxic food contaminants are produced by various filamentous fungi species that are ubiquitous in nature, however, favourable climatic conditions in the tropics favour their proliferation in these regions. Africa, by virtue of its location along the equator makes it highly accommodative to proliferation of mycotoxigenic fungi species, as such, it is the most affected of all the continents. Other factors such as poverty, and climate change further complicates the mycotoxin situation on the continent. Economic impact due to mycotoxin contamination in Africa is thus alarming. The effects of mycotoxins can in fact be felt in the overall health of humans and animals, sustainable development, food security and safety, damage to the African agricultural export brand, negatively impacting Africa's self-sustainability and increased dependence on foreign aid, not excluding high cost of research, mitigation and regulation of the prevalence of these toxins in African countries. This book chapter presents an exhaustive appraisal of the socio-economic impact of mycotoxins on Africa. Our observations herein are expected to stimulate policy makers, as well as, all stakeholders along the food supply chain to identify critical areas of collaboration and strengthen alliances in order to ameliorate the effects of these toxicants on the continent of Africa, and the world at large.

Keywords: mycotoxins, socio-economic impact, Africa, fungi, immunosuppression, hepatotoxic, socio-economic impact, health impact

1. Introduction

Globally, the consumption of contaminated foods accentuates a clear food security threat, and the central elements leading to contamination are microorganisms, specifically, fungi, which produce low-molecular weight toxic secondary metabolites known as mycotoxins. About 25% of the global food and feed output is contaminated by mycotoxins, which negatively affects human and animal health, productivity, livelihood, household security, income and causes significant economic losses [1]. Very often, contamination of agricultural commodities by mycotoxins results from a cumulative process, which begins from pre-harvest through post-harvest stage and continues throughout the entire food production chain [2]. Some factors that drive mycotoxin contamination along the African food and feed chain are the mid and hot tropical climates that are favourable growth conditions for fungi, food shortages, ignorance of the cause and implications of mycotoxins, food dumping and adulteration of foods with mouldy agricultural products as well as inadequate regulatory mechanisms [3, 4].

A recent investigation on the mycotoxin issue across the entire continent of Africa led by Professor Sheila Okoth of the University of Nairobi (Kenya) and commissioned by the Technical Centre for Agricultural and Rural Cooperation (CTA) in conjunction with Partnership for Aflatoxin Control in Africa (PACA), confirmed and re-affirmed the seriousness of the mycotoxin issue [5, 6]. Economic losses arising from mycotoxicosis in Africa are alarming; losses incurred by developed nations are usually trade-related, whereas Africa tends to incur both economic losses and additional costs related to health challenges. This immense socio-economic impact of mycotoxins threatens the UN's sustainable development goal of improving nutrition, achieving food security and attaining a healthy agro-economic growth [6]. Often, socio-economic impact of mycotoxin contamination in Africa can be measured through reduced food availability, specifically amongst the rural poor, regulatory rejections of goods mainly at ports of exit, reduced market value of contaminated produce in domestic markets, decreased marketability of crops, forced alternative uses, increased livestock and human diseases, as well as mortality. Moreover, this impact should not exclude the high cost of research and regulatory activities aimed at reducing health risks because of the existence of causal relationships between mycotoxins and their impact on health. It is also overwhelming that in Africa, an annual cost of over USD 750 million is been accrued to aflatoxin (AF) contamination of crops, while the European Union (EU) regulation of AFs reportedly costs food exporters an estimated USD 670 million yearly [7]. Misdiagnosis, poor infrastructures, undependable and inconsistent data amongst other factors make it difficult to account for the additional and indirect costs associated with mycotoxin exposure in Africa. If the scale of economic and health impact of mycotoxin contamination is well understood, it will hasten policy makers towards imposing regulations and supporting affected populations. This chapter discusses on some pertinent socio-economic impacts of mycotoxin contamination in Africa.

2. Common mycotoxins in Africa and associated factors that facilitate their prevalence

Mycotoxins are secondary metabolites produced by filamentous fungi, especially those members within the *Aspergillus, Penicillium, Fusarium* and *Alternaria* genera, and notable for their toxigenicity and disease-causing effects amongst humans and animals. Different studies on mycotoxins since the discovery of AF in early 1960s have led to the identification of over 300 mycotoxins, few of which have received significant attention due to their health and economic importance.

2.1. Common mycotoxins in Africa

From an African context, the major mycotoxins of significance in terms of health and the economy are the AFs, fumonisins (FBs), ochratoxins (OTs), trichothecenes (THs) and the zearalenones (ZEAs). This is equally relative to their widespread occurrence in major food and feed commodities, aggravated by favourable climatic conditions in the continent. Of all the several occurring mycotoxins, the AFs are considered the most important. This is particularly associated with its prevalence in commodities and potency of aflatoxin B_1 (AFB_1), an AF form known to be the most noxious naturally occurring carcinogen. They have thus received substantial attention as compared to other mycotoxins as they frequently contaminate food and feed commodities in Africa [8]. Though there are about 20 different identified forms of these AFs [9], those of significant and economic importance are AFB_1, aflatoxin B_2 (AFB_2), aflatoxin G_1 (AFG_1) and aflatoxin G_2 (AFG_2). Equally important are also aflatoxins M_1 (AFM_1) and M_2 (AFM_2), which are hydroxylated metabolites of AFB_1 and AFB_2, respectively [10]. FBs, particularly fumonisin B_1 (FB_1), have been classified as a group 2B carcinogen by the International Agency for Research on Cancer (IARC) [11], and is highly prevalent in African staples such as maize, millet and sorghum [12]. The OTs are isocoumarin derivatives, occurring as ochratoxin A (OTA), B (OTB), C (OTC), D (OTD) and their methyl and ethyl esters [13]. Similar to FB_1, OTA is a prevalent toxin, classified as a Group 2B potential carcinogen to human [11]. The THs, which are tetracyclic sesquiterpenes with an epoxy-ring [12, 14], are divided into type A consisting of T-2 and HT-2 toxins and type B with deoxynivalenol (DON) and nivalenol (NIV), the most important representatives [12]. Zearalenone (ZEA) and its hydroxylated derivatives α- and β- zearalenone (α-ZEA and β-ZEA) are lactone derivatives commonly found in food commodities [15]. It has been reported that ZEA usually co-occurs with one or more of the THs, because of the ability of its producing fungi to synthesize more than one mycotoxin [16]. The occurrence of modified and emerging forms of these mycotoxins including 3-acetyldeoxynivalenol (3-ADON), 15-acetyldeoxynivalenol (15-ADON), beauvericin (BEA), the enniatins (ENNs) and moniliformin (MON) have also been reported in African commodities [12]. The prevalence of these mycotoxins in African food crops have been reviewed extensively in literature [17–20], and can be strongly associated with a number of factors which are discussed in the next section.

2.2. Factors that facilitate the prevalence of mycotoxins in Africa

The prevalence of mycotoxins in African food and feed commodities have been well documented in literature, and major factors that contribute to this have been identified as climate change, poverty, limited/lack of awareness, pro-regulation and legislation, poor agricultural practices, amongst others. Climate change has in fact been proposed as probably the most serious environmental issue facing our planet [21], and Africa has been the most affected. In fact, 2016 was identified as the hottest year in about a century, and accordingly, a manifestation of this was the 2016 *El-nino* drought episode of Southern Africa, which resulted in agricultural losses amounting to millions of US dollars (US$). Such imbalances, drastic changes in rainfall, temperature and CO_2 patterns could increase the risk of pathogen migration and influence colonization of crops by mycotoxigenic fungal genera [22]. Since mycotoxin production is climate dependent, changes in climatic conditions have been suggested and proven to lead to possible drastic modifications in fungal population and attendant mycotoxin production [23, 24]. These would not only favour the emergence of new mycotoxigenic fungal strains, but also attendant mycotoxin production in agricultural commodities.

Africa is the poorest continent in the world [25]. Nearly one in five people living in Africa is undernourished and/or go hungry, the highest prevalence of such in the world [26]. This can have a huge significance on the quality of food commodities consumed in Africa. There are limited resources to adopt relevant technologies/systems to control mycotoxins proliferation, and in dire need for food and "quenching" hunger, the quality and safety of food ingested is totally irrelevant (even though visibly contaminated). Under such circumstances, having food is much more vital and subsequently prioritized. Further to this, limited public awareness on the mycotoxins issue has been identified as a critical factor on the prevalence of mycotoxins in Africa. Knowledge is power. The available information on the incidence, public health importance, prevention and control of mycotoxins in many African countries is still grossly lacking, with no indication that such will be addressed anytime soon. Equally important is the lack of appropriate mechanisms to promote and educate consumers on the harmful effects of mycotoxins, good agricultural practices and post-harvest handling of commodities. Due to all these factors, the issue of mycotoxins on the continent has remained infamously persistent, with attendant grave implications. The next section of this chapter discusses in detail the socio-economic impact of these fungal pollutants on the African continent.

3. Socio-economic impact of mycotoxin contamination in Africa

Mycotoxin contamination have contributed significantly to the elusive sustainable development in Africa. The ever daunting and manifest challenges to food safety and security, good health and economic empowerment are all undisputable evidences to this fact.

3.1. Impact of mycotoxins on human and animal health in Africa

3.1.1. Impact of mycotoxins on human health in Africa

The most significant impact of mycotoxin contamination in Africa has been shown to be on human health. A World Bank report in 1993 observed that the various health problems modulated by exposure to mycotoxins accounted for up to 40% of lost disability-adjusted life years (DALYs) [27], and it is no doubt that Africa is the most affected. In 2004, an outbreak caused by food poisoning with AFs occurred in Kenya, where 317 cases of illness were reported and 68 of the persons were children below the age of 5 and 90 were from 5 to 15 years. In this incidence, at least 123 deaths were recorded [28–30]. In sub-Saharan Africa, about 250,000 deaths are caused by hepatocellular carcinoma annually and this can be linked to risk factors such as AFs and high prevalence of hepatitis B [31]. AF contamination in groundnuts and maize in Nigeria contributed to 7761 liver cancer cases, which results in a total burden of 100,965 DALYs [32]. In 2014, due to AF contamination, about 3334 cases of hepatocellular carcinoma was calculated in Tanzania, 95% of which ended as deaths resulting to a loss of 96,686 DALYs [33].

Based on several studies in Southern Africa, AFs contamination have been strongly linked with child undernutrition, increased mortality and morbidity due to their negative effect on micronutrient absorption and immune function [34]. In addition to these, immune disruption by AFs may aggravate health impacts of principal diseases plaguing Africa such as malaria, kwashiorkor and HIV/AIDS [35]. In Nigeria, posthumous autopsy of infants who suffered from kwashiorkor showed a significant level of AFs in their brains, because of consumption of contaminated maize based gruel [36]. According to Jolly *et al.* [37], high levels of AFB_1 and acute aflatoxicosis symptoms were found within Ghanaian population that also had abnormal liver function and high level of HBV infections. Turner *et al.* [38] reported decreased levels of secretory immunoglobulin A (IgA) in Gambian children exposed to AFs. In Kenya, the mean birthweight of the children of women exposed to AFs prenatally was lesser than that of those who had not been similarly exposed [39].

In the Gambia, maternal dietary intake was indicated to be an important factor in carcinogenic-induced damage in the unborn baby, due to a highly significant correlation between AF-albumin adduct levels in the mothers venous and respective cord sera [40]. In the same country, children with reduced level of salivary Secretory Immunoglobulin A (sIgA) have been linked with exposure to AFs [38]. The consumption of FBs contaminated maize have been correlated to the high incidence of oesophageal cancer in parts of South Africa [41] and Malawi [42]. According to Ferlay *et al.* [42], Malawi has the highest prevalence rate (24.2 per 100,000 persons) of oesophageal cancer in the world. ZEA as a naturally occurring endocrine-disrupting chemical has been implicated in the manifestations of gynecomastia with testicular atrophy in rural males in Southern Africa [43]. In 1977 to 1978 an outbreak of ergotism occurred in Wollo, Ethiopia where 140 persons were affected, four children lost both or at least one leg and the mortality as high as 34% [44]. In North Africa, particularly Tunisia and Egypt, cases of human nephropathies have been strongly associated with elevated exposure to OTA and outbreaks of ochratoxicosis, *i.e.*, illness due to ochratoxin exposure [45–47]. Alpha-ZEA has been implicated as a potential risk factor for breast cancer in Tunisia [48]. Likewise, high levels of OTA in Moroccan foods and other agricultural commodities have been linked to some chronic illnesses [49, 50]. **Table 1** shows some other mycotoxins and the toxic effects they provoke on human health. Further studies are required to establish the association between other poorly investigated diseases and dietary exposure to other mycotoxins (emerging, modified and multiple mycotoxins).

Though tremendously difficult to estimate in Africa, the net monetarized impact of mycotoxins on human health in Africa [including physical pain, death (in severe cases), temporary or permanent impairment, loss of productivity, costs of diagnosis, treatment, hospitalization

Mycotoxins	Toxic effects	Reference
Ergot alkaloids	Ergotism: central nervous system disorder, gastrointestinal symptoms, & gangrene	[51]
Citrinin	Hepatonephrotoxic	[51]
Cyclopiazonic acid	Weight loss, diarrhoea, nausea, necrosis, & convulsion	[51]
Patulin	Genotoxic, teratogenic, carcinogenic, & acute toxicity to kidney	[51]
Sterigmatocystin	Carcinogenic, & hepatotoxic	[51]
Rubratoxin	Liver damage, nephrotoxic, & haemorrhage	[51]
Gliotoxin	Neurological syndrome, & immunosuppressive	[51]
Moniliformin	Acutely toxic, & cardiac impairment	[51]
Fumitremorgen	Tremors, & convulsion	[51]
AFs	Carcinogenic, & immunosuppressive	[52]
OTs	Mutagenic, carcinogenic, & nephrotoxic	[53–56]
FBs	Carcinogenic, nephrotoxic, hepatotoxic, immunosuppressive, atherogenic, & embryotoxic	[57, 58]
DON	Immunosuppressive, immunostimulative, & causes fertility problems	[59–62]
ZEAs	Infertility, reduced milk production, vaginal secretions, & vaginitis	[63, 64]
T2-toxin	Cardiovascular defects, gastroenteritis, & alimentary toxic aleukia	[65, 66]

Table 1. Mycotoxins and their toxic effects on human health (adapted from Capriotti ***et al.***) [51].

and health care (morbidity), cost of anxiety, pain, misdiagnosis, suffering and reduced life quality etc.] could be enormous, and demanding on national budget. A case in point, a study conducted in Gambia observed that diseases consistent with mycotoxin exposure (in particular Hepatitis B and its associated medical complications) results in a total monetized DALY worth over 94 million US$ of GDP, which equals 9.4% of the nation's GDP. This is a huge loss to the health of the populace and country [67]. Similarly, in Senegal, the cumulative cost in terms of health due to AFs is estimated at no less than 92 million US$ of the nation's GDP [67]. In 2014 in Tanzania, the economic impact (in monetary terms) of AFs was estimated between 6 million and 264 million US$ due to the resultant health impact [33].

3.1.2. *Impact of mycotoxins on animal health in Africa*

Very little work has been done on the health impact of mycotoxins on animals in Africa. This is understandable as the health effects and losses in animals (such as feeding efficiency, infertility, meat, milk and egg quality losses, susceptibility to diseases etc.) are subtler to decipher. Moreover, in Africa, people have limited resources and may prioritize the care of humans above the 'waste of resources' on animals. To this effect, when mouldy cereals are too bad to be consumed, they are usually not disposed, but blended with non-mouldy ones and used as animal feed, or in some cases fed directly to the animals. However, monogastric farm animals such as poultry, swine and dogs are at particular high risk, because their basal diet (feed) is made up of cereals [68]. These animals also lack reservoir that harbours microorganisms that can break down secondary metabolites of fungi before they are absorbed into the intestine. In South Africa, there have been two episodes of aflatoxicosis (illness resulting from AFs) amongst dogs through the consumption of contaminated dog food. The first occurred in 1987 where 10 cases of fatality were reported, and histopathological evaluation revealed chronic symptoms of necrosis, bile duct proliferation, hepatocellular fatty degeneration, fibroplasia etc. were observed [69]. The second episode occurred in 2011, where over 220 dogs died and several others were affected in the Gauteng province. Subsequent clinical examinations revealed that the dogs were exposed to highly contaminated feed (with levels of AFs ranging from 5 μg/kg and 4946 μg/kg), which is well above regulatory limits [70]. In addition to AFs, other mycotoxins such as FB_1, ZEA, and OTA were all later implicated in this outbreak [71]. Mwanza *et al.* [72] evaluated the productivity and general health of domesticated animals in Limpopo Province of South Africa in relation to fungi and mycotoxin contamination, the results revealed that these animals were at risk to mycotoxin contamination which possibly plays an important role in abortions, low productivity, chronic and acute diseases, as well as reduced immunity in these animals, which are similar effects often seen in other rural communities in the country, as well as other parts of Africa, however, no clinical investigation is usually conducted to determine the possible causes of such illness/effects [72].

3.2. Impact of mycotoxins on food security in Africa

The CTA has clearly alarmed that mycotoxins significantly threatens achieving food security and safety in Africa, which is one of the UN's sustainable development goals [5]. Food supplies are limited and often of poor quality, with mycotoxins proliferation frequently implicated as the culprit. About 35% of global food and feed produce is contaminated by mycotoxins. The attendant food losses/wastages is in the ranks of 1 billion metric tons annually [73–75], and there is little doubt that majority of these losses come from Africa. In a continent where about 60% of the populace are farmers (mainly at a subsistence level), and majority of households relay on their homegrown food for survival, these statistics on mycotoxins are disturbing. The eminent reality of global warming further complicates the situation as Africa is the continent that is most affected due to its position at the equator. A recent study predicts that fungal pathogens and pests are proliferating at a rate of 5–6 km annually from the equator to polar regions of the earth [76]. Drought and plant stress makes crops more susceptible to diseases and fungal attack, and consequently increases mycotoxin contamination, which reduces crop quality and yield, as well as decreases in livestock productivity, disease tolerance and fertility. Moreover, adaptation of known mycotoxigenic fungal species to climate change conditions could result in a more aggressive and invasive behaviour of the fungi leading to colonization of new territories, increased production of mycotoxins, and perhaps the potential of producing entirely new mycotoxins, which poses a significant threat to food security, safety and health in Africa and other developing countries [76–78].

3.3. Impact of mycotoxins on trade and damage to the African agricultural export market brand

Mycotoxins affect trade in Africa majorly by reducing the value of commodities offered for sale. Reduced value can manifest at different trade levels through the lowering of prices, inspection cost, disposal, rejection of lots or treatment of lots at additional cost prior to sale, compensation in case of claims and cost of sampling and analysis along the value chain. Not less than 2.3 million bags of maize were found unsuitable for marketing (as well as consumption) during the outbreak of aflatoxicosis in Kenya from 2004 to 2006 [79]. Following another AF alert in Kitui,

Kenya in 2009, it was reported that maize prices dropped by half from 1800 to 900 Kenyan shillings [79]. The enforcement of regulatory standards primarily by developed nations which are the main destinations of African agricultural export commodities have resulted in a more critical situation for the African agricultural trade [52, 80]. EU regulation of mycotoxins was expected to reduce African export of nuts, cereals, oil seeds and dried fruits by 64%, reportedly costing 670 million US$ yearly [81]. Between 2000 and 2014, the cumulative economic loss on domestic and international trade in Gambia was about 23 million US$, which amounts to a yearly loss of about 1.52 million US$ [67]. The International Institute of Tropical Agriculture (IITA) [82] reported an annual loss of 1.2 billion US$ on a global scale due to AF contamination and established that 38% of this loss (450 million US$) is incurred by African nations.

Another major socio-economic impact of mycotoxins on Africa is the damage to the African agricultural tradename. Brand in general terms can be described as an intangible and invaluable feature that distinguishes an entity from its competitors, and comprises expectations, imaginations, emotions and loyalty by the customers [83]. As a matter of fact, in the field of accounting, it is regarded as the most valuable asset on the balance sheet [84, 85]. Damage to brand can have a significant and enduring (and in some cases irredeemable) impact on subsequent business performance, productivity, reputation, financial gains and business prospects. Unfortunately, the mycotoxin issue has caused significant damage to African food and agricultural trade brand, particularly in the export market. Some of the consequences can be observed in the lack of trust for African food/feed commodities, 'redundant scrutiny' (which may result in transaction delays and perhaps more food spoilage), rejections, etc. A case in point was the significant levels of AFs in groundnuts exported from Africa to Europe in 2007 [86], leading to the serious concern about the future of such and other exports from the African continent.

In 2000, 57 cases of border refusal of African exports to the EU were recorded but these cases have increased over the years and as at 2012, 525 cases were recorded [87]. More specifically, from 2002 to 2008, 130 export rejections from Egypt, 90 from Nigeria, 91 from Ghana, 5 from Morocco and 1 from Tunisia were recorded due to mycotoxin contamination [88]. Also in 2008, Rwanda suffered border rejections of sorghum, maize, soybean flour, destined to United Kingdom due to AFs contamination [89]. Between 2007 and 2012, 13 consignments of groundnut and groundnut related products from Nigeria were also rejected by the EU [90]. The National Agency for Food and Drug Administration (NAFDAC) of Nigeria reported that up to 42 semi-processed and processed food products of Nigeria origin destined for the European Union where rejected in 2015 and 2016 for failing to meet standards [91]. Twenty-eight of these items were destroyed, 6 subjected to official detention, 6 withdrawn from consumers and from the market, and 9 were re-dispatched [91]. Based on data from European Commission Rapid Alert System (RASFF), 35% of food/feed commodities rejections by the EU borders in 2014 were due to mycotoxin contamination at levels above the EU legislative limits [76]. It should be noted that the cost of a rejected food shipment is significant (about 10,000 US$ per lot in demurrage fees) even if the lot can be returned to the country attempting to export [92].

3.4. Impact of mycotoxins on national budget due to mitigation costs

Some African countries have started to set up interventions to reduce the prevalence of mycotoxins in their jurisdiction, however, most of these interventions have high cost implication with regards to their design and implementation. In 2014, the Economic Community for

West African States (ECOWAS) in collaboration with the African Union's PACA and other stakeholders developed the "ECOWAS Aflatoxin Control Action Plan (ECOACAP)" which identified key actionable strategic interventions in order to combat the prevalence of AFs across ECOWAS member States. Policy 4.3 SO3 of this plan recommended that ECOWAS member states increase budgetary allocations and investments to at least 1% of national GDP for the development and enforcement of AFs control efforts [67]. An annual cost of 7.5 million US$ was calculated by member states of the African Groundnut Council (Mali, Nigeria, Gambia, Sudan, Niger and Senegal) for the implementation of an AF contamination reduction program [90]. The Maize Trust, an initiative principally funded by the government of South Africa, spends over 4 million US$ per annum on funding projects directly targeted at improving the South African maize industry, and one of the outlined key objectives is to combat mycotoxins in South African maize [93]. Details of other interventions sponsored by other African governments can be found in the PACA report [94].

3.5. Impact of mycotoxins on Africa's self-sustainability and increased dependence on foreign aid

Africa has been caught in a vicious circle of the cause and effects of mycotoxin contamination and poverty. Mycotoxins aggravates poverty, and due to poverty, many African countries lack the resources to sponsor effective mycotoxin research and mitigation interventions, which further worsens the situation on the continent. As such, majority of the mycotoxin projects conducted on the continent are sponsored by external sources, hence, increasing Africa's dependence of foreign aid. For instance, the US government via the Feed the Future (FTF) initiative of the United States Agency for International Development (USAID) Bureau for Food Security budgeted 2–5 million US$ per year in 2010, and 15–20 million US$ per year in 2014, for AF-specific researches in African countries and developing countries in other continents [95]. Ghent University, Belgium sponsored an international thematic network 'Mytox-South' established in 2017, with an initial approved funding of 600,000 EUR. This intends to build/strengthen the human capacity of researchers from the Southern Hemisphere, leveraging on infrastructure and expertise at Ghent University in order to combat the mycotoxin problem and associated food security and safety issues at global level [96]. The Standards and trade development facility (STDF) sponsored a six month project on strengthening AF control in the Republic of Malawi through the Malawi Programme for Aflatoxin Control (MAPAC) with a budget of 46,265 thousand US$ [97]. Details on other foreign mycotoxin interventions in Africa worth millions of US$ can be found from these sources [94, 98, 99].

Interestingly, even the private sector has not been left out. Recently, the spotlight has turned on strengthening coalitions with the private sector, while leveraging on the efforts of different actors for effective management of mycotoxins in Africa. In October 2016, PACA and CTA convened a roundtable event in Entebbe, Uganda to identify concrete areas of collaboration and evaluate avenues for effective public-private sector partnership and engagement in the common agenda for tackling mycotoxin prevalence. CEOs and other representatives from various private establishments such as Cereal Millers' Association—Kenya, AFRI-Nut—Malawi, CTA, Meds For Kids—Haiti, GrainPro—East Africa, PACA, USAID, Nestlé—West Africa, various Women's organisations in Zimbabwe and Uganda, were in attendance, amongst others [5, 6].

4. Commitment to research and awareness as effective tools in mitigating the impact of mycotoxins in Africa

Mycotoxicology research is an important component of mycotoxin management. Particularly in Africa, more research needs to be done in order to establish safe limits and guard against potential health hazards. Availability of stringent scientific data provides the basis for government regulatory bodies to assess the risk of exposure, as well as, establish/enforce or reassess regulatory limits for mycotoxins [52, 100]. For example, from central African countries, there is hardly any information on mycotoxins. This may be due to ignorance on the mycotoxin issue, poverty, lack of research facilities and skills/manpower in these countries [17]. In a recent study by Adekoya *et al.* [101], the perceived understanding, practices and health risks related to fungal and mycotoxin contamination amongst fermented food sellers was evaluated. It was observed that up to 98% of respondents were unaware of mycotoxin contamination [101]. Elsewhere, findings by Changwa [102] in South Africa indicated that there are several knowledge gaps on the mycotoxin issue, such as causes of mycotoxins, health implications, prevention and control of mycotoxins, which corroborates the observation of Adekoya *et al.* [101]. In a recent round-table discussion on future directions in research facilitated by the European Horizon2020 project, MycoKey, it was agreed that forging partnerships between scientists and appropriately-placed communication experts constitutes a critical avenue for creating awareness and communicating risks, while maintaining overall confidence in the quality and safety along the food supply chain [103].

Despite all said, it must be acknowledged that mycotoxin research in Africa has yielded fruitful and positive results. While some of these studies were funded by governments in the continent, many are equally funded by research organizations and governments of other developed nations. For example, researchers at IITA and the University of Ibadan, in partnership with the Agriculture Research Service (ARS) of the United States Department of Agriculture developed a natural, safe and affordable solution to the problem of AF called "Aflasafe™", intended for use by groundnut and maize farmers. The product which contains non-toxigenic strains of *A. flavus*, is reported to be able to reduce AF levels in maize by 80–100%, and together with other good agricultural practices will increase the crop value by at least 25%, as well as improve the health of children and women [104, 105]. Due to the immense success of Aflasafe™, expansion of the biocontrol research reached Ghana, Tanzania, Burkina Faso, Senegal, Kenya, Mali, and Zambia [105]. AflaSTOP is another project which started in 2012, aimed at identifying the most effective, efficient, low-cost, innovative storage and drying technology to combat AF contamination, and other post-harvest losses in Kenya, Tanzania and Rwanda [106]. The Aflasafe™ and Aflastop projects together with other mycotoxin projects described herein [95, 105] cost about 15–20 million US$ in 2014 and 2–5 million US$ in 2010, sponsored by the US Government under the Feed the Future (FTF)—USAID Bureau for Food Security [95, 105].

Last year 2017, Ethiopia farmers/researchers supported by Ethiopia's Agricultural Transformation Agency, was able to produce and market much of the 27 tons of new, disease-resistant wheat seed, in direct response to an annual attack of rapidly-evolving fungal diseases that can infect their locally grown crops worth as much as 200 million US$ [107]. Elsewhere, several African scientists are working on a project aimed at reduction of AF contamination via RNA interference (RNAi) in peanut plants. Three peanut varieties endemic to Africa are currently been genetically transformed at Kenyatta University in Nairobi, Kenya, by means of RNAi molecular constructs. Many of the African scientists involved in the project have been trained hands-on at the National Peanut Research Laboratory (NPRL) in Dawson, Georgia [99]. At the University of Johannesburg and Stellenbosch University both in South Africa, microbial means of degrading and detoxifying mycotoxins have also been proposed as a possible way of reducing/eliminating mycotoxins in food [108–110].

Previously, much of research was focused on producing enough food to meet the teaming population of the world, however, it is becoming more obvious that reducing food spoilage/loss and contamination could be a more efficient approach towards addressing issues of food security particularly in Africa. As a way forward, research objectives should be prioritized to ensure a positive impact for public health, food safety and security and economic development. Recently, a global initiative has been launched, The Mycotox Charter, which provides a global platform for the various players along the food supply chain to commit to the mycotoxin cause, by means of a globally applicable statement and clearly outlined principles and practices targeted at reducing mycotoxin contamination in food and feed and associated health problems [111]. It is hoped that such an initiative will achieve its objectives in addressing these problems linked to mycotoxins.

5. Conclusion

The impact of mycotoxins on Africa has been and is still illustrious. Limited knowledge/awareness, poverty, bad governance and climatic conditions have further aggravated this unfortunate situation. Africa is the largest continent in the world and the most plagued by the mycotoxin menace. Despite the notoriously incessant occurrence and exceptionally high levels of mycotoxins reported in dietary food for humans and animals, and the associated lethal consequences, regulation for their control and management is significantly limited in this part of the world. It has been projected that between 2015 and 2050, the population of Africa will increase by 1.3 billion people. In fact, according to the UN, the population of Nigeria alone is projected to surpass that of the entire US by 2050. This teaming population puts immense pressure on the already scarce food resources on the continent. More compelling is the fact that Africa's population is comprised mainly of the younger age (with two-fifths between the ages of 0–14 years, and one-fifth in the age bracket to 15–24 years), where good food and health plays a critical role in the overall development of individuals. As such, the proliferation and widespread effect of mycotoxins in Africa is of great concern. The eminent reality of climate change is also looming steadily with Africa at the epicentre. Biodiversification of fungi due to adaptation to climate change leads to threats of newer mycotoxins or more of existing ones. In order to stay aligned with the UN's sustainable development goals (particularly goal No. 2: end hunger, achieve food security and improved nutrition and promote sustainable agriculture), a concerted effort is needed to adequately address the issue of mycotoxin in Africa and other developing countries of the world. Critical areas to concentrate efforts include development of efficient and cost-effective intervention strategies, public awareness, strengthening research and human capacity development as well as harmonizing and enforcing regulations.

Acknowledgements

This work was financially supported via the Global Excellence and Stature (GES) Fellowship of the University of Johannesburg granted to the main author (S. Gbashi), as well as, the South African National Research Foundation (NRF).

Author details

Sefater Gbashi[1*], Ntakadzeni Edwin Madala[2], Sarah De Saeger[3], Marthe De Boevre[3], Ifeoluwa Adekoya[1], Oluwafemi Ayodeji Adebo[1] and Patrick Berka Njobeh[1]

*Address all correspondence to: sefatergbashi@gmail.com

1 Department of Biotechnology and Food Technology, Faculty of Science, University of Johannesburg, Doornfontein Campus, Gauteng, South Africa

2 Department of Biochemistry, School of Mathematical and Natural Sciences, University of Venda, Thohoyandou, South Africa

3 Laboratory of Food Analysis, Department of Bioanalysis, Ghent University, Ghent, Belgium

References

[1] Enyiukwu DN, Awurum AN, Nwaneri JA. Mycotoxins in stored agricultural products: Implications to food safety and health and prospects of plant-derived pesticides as novel approach to their management. Greener Journal of Microbiology and Antimicrobials. 2014;**2**(3):32-48

[2] Wilson DM, Abramson D. Mycotoxins. In: Sauer DB, editor. Storage of Cereal Grains and their Products. Saint Paul, Minnesota: American Association of Cereal Chemists; 1992. pp. 341-391

[3] Njobeh PB, Olotu I. The socio-economic impact of mycotoxin contamination in Africa. In: Proceedings of the 1st MYCOKEY International Conference. Global Mycotoxin Reduction in the Food and Feed Chain. September 11-14, 2017. Ghent, Belgium: Toxins; 2017

[4] Mejía-Teniente L, Chapa-Oliver AM, Vazquez-Cruz MA, Torres-Pacheco I, Guevara-González RG. Aflatoxins biochemistry and molecular biology - biotechnological approaches for control in crops. In: Torres-Pacheco I, editor. Aflatoxins – Detection, Measurement and Control. Rijeka, Croatia: InTech; 2011. pp. 317-354

[5] CTA. Mitigating the consequences of aflatoxin in Africa - what role for the private sector? Agricultural policies - technical Centre for Agricultural and Rural Cooperation ACP-EU (CTA) in conjunction with the Partnership for Aflatoxin Control in Africa (PACA); 2016.

(Online) Retrieved December 20, 2017, from http://www.cta.int/en/article/2016-10-21/mitigating-the-consequences-of-aflatoxin-in-africa.html

[6] AUC-PACA and CTA. Engaging the private sector for aflatoxin control in Africa. Concept note. Technical Centre for Agricultural and Rural Cooperation ACP-EU (CTA) in conjunction with the Partnership for Aflatoxin Control in Africa (PACA), Entebbe, Uganda; 2016. (Online) Retrieved December 20, 2017, from http://www.cta.int/images/PACA_CTA_Concept Note_Engaging the Private Sector for Aflatoxin Controlv2_JAF CTA_080916.pdf

[7] Udomkun P, Wiredu AN, Nagle M, Bandyopadhyay R, Müller J, Vanlauwe B. Mycotoxins in sub Saharan Africa: Present situation, socio-economic impact, awareness, and outlook. Food Control. 2017;**72**:110-122

[8] Makun HA, Dutton MF, Njobeh PB, Gbodi TA, Ogbadu GH. Aflatoxin contamination in foods and feeds: A special focus on Africa. In: Ayman AE, editor. Trends in Vital Food and Control Engineering. Rijeka, Croatia: InTech; 2012. pp. 187-234

[9] Marin S, Ramos AJ, Cano-Sancho G, Sanchis V. Mycotoxins: Occurrence, toxicology, and exposure assessment. Food and Chemical Toxicology. 2013;**60**:218-237

[10] Dors GC, Caldas SS, Feddern V, Bemvenuti RH, dos Santos Hackbart HC, de Souza MM, dos Santos Oliveira M, Garda-Buffon J, Primel EG, Badiale-Furlong E. Aflatoxins: Contamination, analysis and control. In: Guevara-Gonzalez RG, editor. Aflatoxins-Biochemistry and Molecular Biology. Rijeka, Croatia: InTech; 2011. pp. 415-438

[11] IARC. Some traditional herbal medicines, some mycotoxins, naphthalene and styrene. In: Monographs on the Evaluation of Carcinogenic Risks to Humans (Vol. 82). Lyon, France: International Agency for Research on Cancer (IARC) - World Health Organization. Monographs on the evaluation of carcinogenic risks to humans; 2002

[12] Chilaka CA, De Boevre M, Atanda OO, De Saeger S. The status of Fusarium mycotoxins in sub-Saharan Africa: A review of emerging trends and post-harvest mitigation strategies towards food control. Toxins. 2017;**9**(1):1-37

[13] Haschek Haschek WM, Voss KA, Beasley VR. Selected mycotoxins affecting animal and human health. In: Handbook of Toxicologic Pathology. 2nd ed. Vol. 1. San Diego, California: Academic Press; 2002. pp. 645-699

[14] Mbundi L, Gallar-Ayala H, Khan MR, Barber JL, Losada S, Busquets R. Advances in the analysis of challenging food contaminants: Nanoparticles, bisphenols, mycotoxins, and brominated flame retardants. Advances in Molecular Toxicology. 2014;**8**:35-105

[15] Gratz SW. Do Plant-bound masked Mycotoxins contribute to toxicity? Toxins. 2017;**9**(3):85

[16] Grenier B, Oswald I. Mycotoxin co-contamination of food and feed: Meta-analysis of publications describing toxicological interactions. World Mycotoxin Journal. 2011;**4**(3):285-313

[17] Darwish WS, Ikenaka Y, Nakayama SM, Ishizuka M. An overview on mycotoxin contamination of foods in Africa. Journal of Veterinary Medical Science. 2014;**76**(6):789-797

[18] Magoha H, Kimanya M, De Meulenaer B, Roberfroid D, Lachat C, Kolsteren P. Risk of dietary exposure to aflatoxins and fumonisins in infants less than 6 months of age in Rombo, northern Tanzania. Maternal and Child Nutrition. 2014;**12**(3):516-527

[19] Cardwell KF. Mycotoxin contamination of foods in Africa: Antinutritional factors. Food and Nutrition Bulletin. 2000;**21**(4):488-492

[20] Misihairabgwi JM, Ezekiel CN, Sulyok M, Shephard GS, Krska R. Mycotoxin contamination of foods in southern Africa: A 10-year review (2007-2016). Critical Reviews in Food Science and Nutrition. 2017:1-16

[21] Paterson RRM, Lima N. How will climate change affect mycotoxins in food? Food Research International. 2010;**43**(7):1902-1914

[22] Magan N, Medina A, Aldred D. Possible climate-change effects on mycotoxin contamination of food crops pre-and postharvest. Plant Pathology. 2011;**60**(1):150-163

[23] Madgwick JW, West JS, White RP, Semenov MA, Townsend JA, Turner JA, Fitt BD. Impacts of climate change on wheat anthesis and fusarium ear blight in the UK. European Journal of Plant Pathology. 2011;**130**(1):117-131

[24] Van der Fels-Klerx HJ, Liu C, Battilani P. Modelling climate change impacts on mycotoxin contamination. World Mycotoxin Journal. 2016;**9**(5):717-726

[25] Chihombori-Quao A. Q & A with AU ambassador to US Arikana Chihombori-Quao. In: Aljazeera. 2017. Retrieved January 31, 2018, from http://www.aljazeera.com/indepth/features/2017/07/qa-au-ambassador-arikana-chihombori-quao-170719090234363.html

[26] Hedden S, Hughes BB, Rothman DS, Markle AJ, Maweni J, Mayaki IA. Ending hunger in Africa: The elimination of hunger and food insecurity on the African continent by 2025: Conditions for success. In: NEPAD Eliminating Hunger Report Summary (Pp. 3-46). Colorado, USA: Frederick S. Pardee Center for International Futures, University of Denver; 2016

[27] Marechera G, Ndwiga J. Farmer perceptions of aflatoxin management strategies in lower eastern Kenya. Journal of Agricultural Extension and Rural Development. 2014;**6**(12):382-392

[28] Lewis L, Onsongo M, Njapau H, Schurz-Rogers H, Luber G, Kieszak S, Nyamongo J, Backer L, Dahiye AM, Misore A, DeCock K, Rubin C. Aflatoxin contamination of commercial maize products during an outbreak of acute aflatoxicosis in eastern and Central Kenya. Environmental Health Perspective. 2005;**113**(12):1763-1767

[29] Azziz-Baumgartner E, Lindblade K, Gieseker K, Rogers HS, Kieszak S, Njapau H, Schleicher R, McCoy LF, Misore A, DeCock K, Rubin C, Slutsker L. Case-control study of an acute aflatoxicosis outbreak, Kenya, 2004. Environmental Health Perspective. 2005;**113**(12):1779-1783

[30] Peraica M, Richter D, Rašić D. Mycotoxicoses in children. Archives of Industrial Hygiene and Toxicology. 2014;**65**(4):347-363

[31] Zain ME. Impact of mycotoxins on humans and animals. Journal of Saudi Chemical Society. 2011;**15**(2):129-144

[32] Atanda O, Ndenn J, Diedhiou P. The economic impact of aflatoxins in West Africa: The case of Nigeria, Gambia and Senegal; 2015. Retrieved February 5, 2018, from http://aflatoxinpartnership.org/uploads/2.3 - Economic impact of aflatoxin in West Africa.pdf

[33] Kimanya ME, Tiisekwa B, Mpolya E. Country and Economic Assessment for Aflatoxin Contamination and Control in Tanzania; a Supplement to the 2012 Report. Tanzania: Arusha; 2012

[34] Katerere DR, Shephard GS, Faber M. Infant malnutrition and chronic aflatoxicosis in southern Africa: Is there a link? International journal of food safety. Nutrition and Public Health. 2008;**1**(2):127-136

[35] Gnonlonfin GJB, Hell K, Adjovi Y, Fandohan P, Koudande DO, Mensah GA, Sanni A, Brimer L. A review on aflatoxin contamination and its implications in the developing world: A sub-Saharan African perspective. Critical Reviews in Food Science and Nutrition. 2013;**53**(4):349-365

[36] Oyelami OA, Maxwell SM, Adelusola KA, Aladekoma TA, Oyelese AO. Aflatoxins in the lungs of children with kwashiorkor and children with miscellaneous diseases in Nigeria. Journal of Toxicology and Environmental Health. 1997;**51**(6):623-628

[37] Jolly PE, Jiang Y, Ellis WO, Awuah RT, Appawu J, Nnedu O, Williams JH. Association between aflatoxin exposure and health characteristics, liver function, hepatitis and malaria infections in Ghanaians. Journal of Nutritional and Environmental Medicine. 2007;**16**(3-4):242-257

[38] Turner PC, Moore SE, Hall AJ, Prentice AM, Wild CP. Modification of immune function through exposure to dietary aflatoxin in Gambian children. Environmental Health Perspectives. 2003;**111**(2):217-220

[39] Hendrickse RG. Of sick turkeys, kwashiorkor, malaria, perinatal mortality, heroin addicts and food poisoning: Research on the influence of aflatoxins on child health in the tropics. Annals of Tropical Paediatrics. 1999;**19**(3):229-235

[40] Wild CP, Rasheed FN, Jawla MFB, Hall AJ, Jansen LAM, Montesano R. In-utero exposure to aflatoxin in West Africa. The Lancet. 1991;**337**(8757):1602

[41] Wagacha JM, Muthomi JW. Mycotoxin problem in Africa: Current status, implications to food safety and health and possible management strategies. International Journal of Food Microbiology. 2008;**124**(1):1-12

[42] Ferlay J, Soerjomataram I, Dikshit R, Eser S. Mortality world-wide. In: Cancer Incidence and Mortality Worldwide: IARC Cancer Base No. 11. 2013

[43] Shephard GS. Impact of mycotoxins on human health in developing countries. Food Additives and Contaminants. 2008;**25**(2):146-151

[44] King B. Outbreak of ergotism in Wollo, Ethiopia. The Lancet. 1979;**313**(8131):1411

[45] Wafa EW, Yahya RS, Sobh MA, Eraky I, El-Baz M, El-Gayar HA, Betbeder AM, Creppy EE. Human ochratoxicosis and nephropathy in Egypt: A preliminary study. Human and Experimental Toxicology. 1998;**17**(2):124-129

[46] Maaroufi K, Achour A, Hammami M, El May M, Betbeder AM, Ellouz F, Creppy EE, Bacha H. Ochratoxin a in human blood in relation to nephropathy in Tunisia. Human and Experimental Toxicology. 1995;**14**(7):609-614

[47] Zaied C, Bouaziz C, Azizi I, Bensassi F, Chour A, Bacha H, Abid S. Presence of ochratoxin a in Tunisian blood nephropathy patients. Exposure level to OTA. Experimental and Toxicologic Pathology. 2011;**63**(7-8):613-618

[48] Belhassen H, Jiménez-Díaz I, Arrebola JP, Ghali R, Ghorbel H, Olea N, Hedili A. Zearalenone and its metabolites in urine and breast cancer risk: A case-control study in Tunisia. Chemosphere. 2015;**128**:1-6

[49] Zinedine A, Mañes J. Occurrence and legislation of mycotoxins in food and feed from Morocco. Food Control. 2009;**20**(4):334-344

[50] Filali A, Betbeder AM, Baudrimont I, Benayada A, Soulaymani R, Creppy EE. Ochratoxin a in human plasma in Morocco: A preliminary survey. Human and Experimental Toxicology. 2002;**21**(5):241-245

[51] Capriotti AL, Caruso G, Cavaliere C, Foglia P, Samperi R, Laganà A. Multiclass mycotoxin analysis in food, environmental and biological matrices with chromatography/mass spectrometry. Mass Spectrometry Reviews. 2012;**31**(4):466-503

[52] Gbashi S, Madala NE, Adebo OA, Piater L, Phoku JZ, Njobeh PB. Subcritical water extraction and its prospects for aflatoxins extraction in biological materials. In: Abdulra'uf LB, editor. Aflatoxin-Control, Analysis, Detection and Health Risks. Rijeka, Croatia: InTech; 2017. pp. 229-250

[53] Clark HA, Snedeker SM. Ochratoxin A: Its cancer risk and potential for exposure. Part B, Critical Reviews. 2006;**9**(3):265-296

[54] Malir F, Ostry V, Pfohl-Leszkowicz A, Malir J, Toman J. Ochratoxin a: 50 years of research. Toxins. 2016;**8**(7):191 (1-49)

[55] Palma N, Cinelli S, Sapora O, Wilson SH, Dogliotti E. Ochratoxin A-induced mutagenesis in mammalian cells is consistent with the production of oxidative stress. Chemical Research in Toxicology. 2007;**20**(7):1031-1037

[56] Pfohl-Leszkowicz A, Manderville RA. Ochratoxin a: An overview on toxicity and carcinogenicity in animals and humans. Molecular Nutrition and Food Research. 2007;**51**(1):61-99

[57] Soriano JM, Dragacci S. Occurrence of fumonisins in foods. Food Research International. 2004;**37**:985-1000

[58] Nair MG. Fumonisins and human health. Annals of Tropical Paediatrics. 1998;**18**:S47-S52

[59] Awad W, Ghareeb K, Böhm J, Zentek J. The toxicological impacts of the fusarium mycotoxin, deoxynivalenol, in poultry flocks with special reference to immunotoxicity. Toxins. 2013;**5**(5):912-925

[60] Bondy GS, Pestka JJ. Immunomodulation by fungal toxins. Journal of Toxicology and Environmental Health, Part B. 2000;**3**(2):109-143

[61] Pinton P, Braicu C, Nougayrede JP, Laffitte J, Taranu I, Oswald IP. Deoxynivalenol impairs porcine intestinal barrier function and decreases the protein expression of claudin-4 through a mitogen-activated protein kinase dependent mechanism. Journal of Nutrition. 2010;**140**(11):1956-1962

[62] Becker C, Reiter M, Pfaffl MW, Meyer HH, Bauer J, Meyer KH. Expression of immune relevant genes in pigs under the influence of low doses of deoxynivalenol (DON). Mycotoxin Research. 2011;**27**(4):287-293

[63] Zinedine A, Soriano JM, Molto JC, Manes J. Review on the toxicity, occurrence, metabolism, detoxification, regulations and intake of zearalenone: An oestrogenic mycotoxin. Food and Chemical Toxicology. 2007;**45**:1-18

[64] Agag BI. Mycotoxins in foods and feeds 3-zearalenone. Assiut University Bulletin for Environmental Researches. 2004;**7**(2):169-176

[65] Yuan G, Wang Y, Yuan X, Zhang T, Zhao J, Huang L, Peng S. T-2 toxin induces developmental toxicity and apoptosis in zebrafish embryos. Journal of Environmental Sciences. 2014;**26**(4):917-925

[66] Semple RL, Frio AS, Hicks PA, Lozare JV. Mycotoxin Prevention and Control in Foodgrains. Italy: Rome; 1989

[67] ECOACAP. Aflatoxin control action plan for ECOWAS member states 2014-2024. ECOWAS Aflatoxin control action plan 2014, 1-35; 2014. Retrieved February 18, 2018 from, http://aflatoxinpartnership.org/uploads/ECOWAS Action Plan- FINAL DRAFT.pdf

[68] Bhat R, Rai RV, Karim AA. Mycotoxins in food and feed: Present status and future concerns. Comprehensive Reviews in Food Science and Food Safety. 2010;**9**(1):57-81

[69] Bastianello SS, Nesbit JW, Williams MC, Lange AL. Pathological findings in a natural outbreak of aflatoxicosis in dogs. The Onderstepoort Journal of Veterinary Research. 1987;**54**(4):635-640

[70] Arnot LF, Duncan NM, Coetzer H, Botha CJ. An outbreak of canine aflatoxicosis in Gauteng Province, South Africa. Journal of the South African Veterinary Association. 2012;**83**(1):1-4

[71] Mwanza M, Ndou RV, Dzoma B, Nyirenda M, Bakunzi F. Canine aflatoxicosis outbreak in South Africa (2011): A possible multi-mycotoxins aetiology. Journal of the South African Veterinary Association. 2013;**84**(1):1-5

[72] Mwanza M. An investigation in South African domesticated animals, their products and related health issues with reference to mycotoxins and fungi. In: Masters Dissertation. South Africa: University of Johannesburg; 2007

[73] Rahmani A, Jinap S, Soleimany F. Qualitative and quantitative analysis of mycotoxins. Comprehensive Reviews in Food Science and Food Safety. 2009;**8**:202-251

[74] Rajani P, Sridevi V, Lakshmi MVVC. A review on biological control of aflatoxin crop contamination. International Journal of Chemical, Environmental and Pharmaceutical Research. 2012;**3**(1):83-86

[75] Schmale DG, Munkvold GP. Mycotoxins in crops: A threat to human and domestic animal health. The Plant Health Instructor. 2009;**3**:340-353

[76] Magan N, Medina A. Mycotoxins, food security and climate change: Do we know enough?; 2016. Retrieved January 10, 2018, from https://microbiologysociety.org/publication/past-issues/fungal-diseases/article/mycotoxins-food-security-and-climate-change-do-we-know-enough-fungal-diseases.html

[77] Magan N, Aldred D, Medina A. Food security, climate change and mycotoxins. Quality Assurance and Safety of Crops and Foods. 2012;**4**(3):145-145

[78] Medina A, Akbar A, Baazeem A, Rodriguez A, Magan N. Climate change, food security and mycotoxins: Do we know enough? Fungal Biology Reviews. 2017;**31**(3):143-154

[79] Marechera G. Estimation of the potential adoption of Aflasafe among smallholder maize farmers in lower eastern Kenya. African Journal of Agriculture and Resource Economics. 2015;**10**(1):72-85

[80] Wu F. Mycotoxin risk assessment for the purpose of setting international regulatory standards. Environmental Science and Technology. 2004;**38**(15):4049-4055

[81] Bankole SA, Adebanjo A. Mycotoxins in food in West Africa: Current situation and possibilities of controlling it. African Journal of Biotechnology. 2003;**2**(9):254-263

[82] IITA. Annual report 2012. International Institute of Tropical Agriculture (IITA) (pp. 14-62). Croydon, UK; 2012. Retrieved on February 18, 2018 from, http://newint.iita.org/wp-content/uploads/2016/04/Annual-Report-2013.pdf

[83] Ghodeswar BM. Building brand identity in competitive markets: A conceptual model. Journal of Product and Brand Management. 2008;**17**(1):4-12

[84] Soler-Labajos N, Jimenez-Zarco AI. Country brand management: Assessing the role of social media in creating the image of Marca Espana (Spain brand). In: Singh A, Duhan P, editors. Managing Public Relations and Brand Image through Social Media. Pennsylvania, USA: Business Science Reference; 2016. pp. 91-92

[85] Sharma MK. Product branding strategy. International Journal of Marketing and Financial Management. 2014;**2**(7):80-86

[86] Unnevehr LJ, Grace D. Tackling aflatoxins: An overview of challenges and solutions. In: Unnevehr LJ, Grace D, editors. Aflatoxins: Finding Solutions for Improved Food Safety, Vision 2020 (P. 2). Washington, DC: International Food Policy Research Institute (IFPRI); 2013

[87] RASFF. Notification details. Rapid alert system for food and feed. European Commission, health and food safety; 2012. Retrieved May 13, 2017, from https://webgate.ec.europa.

eu/rasffwindow/%0Aportal/?event=SearchByKeyword&NewSearch=%0A1&Keywords=egusi

[88] Kareem OI. The European Union sanitary and phytosanitary measures and Africa's exports. In: Global Governance Programme-137. EUI Working Paper RSCAS 2014/98. Italy: San Domenico di Fiesole (FI); 2014

[89] Matsiko F, Kanyange C, Ingabire G, Dusingizimana T, Vasanthakaalam H, Kimonyo A. Detection and quantification of aflatoxin in cassava and maize flour sold in Kigali open markets, Rwanda. International Food Research Journal. 2017;**24**(1):459-464

[90] Atanda O, Makun HA, Ogara IM, Edema M, Idahor KO, Eshiett ME, Oluwabamiwo BF. Fungal and mycotoxin contamination of Nigerian foods and feeds. In: Makun HA, editor. Mycotoxin and Food Safety in Developing Countries. Rijeka, Croatia: InTech; 2013. pp. 1-38

[91] Ogunfuwa I. EU rejects 67 Nigerian foods in two years; 2017. Retrieved January 10, 2018, from http://punchng.com/eu-rejects-67-nigerian-foods-two-years/

[92] Wu F, Liu Y, Bhatnagar D. Cost-effectiveness of aflatoxin control methods: Economic incentives. Toxin Reviews. 2008;**27**(42067):203-225

[93] Du Plessis L. The maize trust: Custodian of the maize industry; 2014. Retrieved February 13, 2018, from http://www.grainsa.co.za/the-maize-trust:-custodian-of-the-maize-industry

[94] PACA. Activities in Africa. The Partnership for Aflatoxin Control in Africa (PACA); 2018. Retrieved February 14, 2018, from http://www.aflatoxinpartnership.org/?q=activities-in-africa

[95] Bowman J, Leslie J, Wu F. How mycotoxins impact agriculture, nutrition and development. USAID Bureau for Food Security. 2012

[96] Mytox-South. MYTOX-SOUTH—An intercontinental partnership striving to solve mycotoxin problems; 2017. Retrieved 20 April 2018 from http://mytoxsouth.org/

[97] Lilongwe M. Advancing collaboration for effective aflatoxin control in Malawi. Malawi Programme for Aflatoxin Control (MAPAC). 2013:1-52

[98] Grace D. Second joint CGIAR meeting on mycotoxins. In: Consultative Group on International Agricultural Research (CGIAR). Naivasha, Kenya. 2013. pp. 3-15. Retrieved February 18, 2018 from, https://a4nh.cgiar.org/files/2013/10/A4NH-aflatoxin-meeting-report-Oct2013.pdf

[99] Arias RS. RNAI Silencing of Aflatoxin Synthesis. Feed the Future Peanut and Mycotoxin Innovation Laboratory. University of Georgia, College of Agricultural and Environmental Sciences; 2016. Retrieved December 28, 2017, from http://www.caes.uga.edu/global/feed-the-future-innovation-labs/peanut-mycotoxin-innovation-lab/Research/USDA201.html

[100] FAO. Worldwide regulations for mycotoxins in food and feed in 2003. Food and Agriculture Organization (FAO) - Food and Nutrition Paper 81. Rome, Italy; 2004

[101] Adekoya I, Njobeh P, Obadina A, Chilaka C, Okoth S, De Boevre M, De Saeger S. Awareness and prevalence of mycotoxin contamination in selected Nigerian fermented foods. Toxins. 2017;**9**(11):363

[102] Changwa R. Quantification of multi-mycotoxins in animal feeds from Gauteng Province using UHPLC-QTOF-MS/MS. In: Masters Dissertation. South Africa: University of Johannesburg; 2017

[103] Leslie JF, Lattanzio V, Audenaert K, Battilani P, Cary J, Chulze SN, De Saeger S, Gerardino A, Karlovsky P, Liao YC, Maragos CM, Meca G, Medina A, Moretti A, Munkvold G, Mulè G, Njobeh P, Pecorelli I, Perrone G, Pietri A, Palazzini JM, Proctor RH, Rahayu ES, Ramírez ML, Samson R, Stroka J, Sulyok M, Sumarah M, Waalwijk C, Zhang Q, Zhang H, Logrieco AF. MycoKey round table discussions of future directions in research on chemical detection methods, genetics and biodiversity of mycotoxins. Toxins. 2018;**10**(3):109

[104] Aflasafe. Aflasafe - safer food in Africa; 2017. Retrieved December 27, 2017, from https://aflasafe.com/aflasafe/

[105] CIMMYT. Tackling Toxins with aflasafeTM. International Maize and Wheat Improvement Center - Centro Internacional de Mejoramiento de Maíz y Trigo (CIMMYT); 2013. Retrieved December 27, 2017, from http://www.cimmyt.org/tackling-toxins-with-aflasafe/

[106] Raimond R. AflaSTOP project identifies the most promising storage options to arrest aflatoxin growth in Kenya, Rwanda and Tanzania. In: SAVE FOOD: Global Initiative on Food Loss and Waste Reduction - Community of Practice on Food Loss Reduction; 2012. Retrieved December 27, 2017, from http://www.fao.org/food-loss-reduction/news/detail/en/c/413664/

[107] Listman M. Ethiopian Farmers Profit from Scaled-up, Fast-Track Production of Disease Resistant Wheat Seed. International Maize and Wheat Improvement Center - Centro Internacional de Mejoramiento de Maíz y Trigo (CIMMYT); 2017. Retrieved December 27, 2018, from http://www.cimmyt.org/ethiopian-farmers-profit-from-scaled-up-fast-track-production-of-disease-resistant-wheat-seed/

[108] Adebo OA, Njobeh PB, Sidu S, Tlou MG, Mavumengwana V. Aflatoxin B_1 degradation by liquid cultures and lysates of three bacterial strains. International Journal of Food Microbiology. 2016;**233**:11-19

[109] Adebo OA, Njobeh PB, Mavumengwana V. Degradation and detoxification of AFB_1 by Staphylocococcus warneri, Sporosarcina sp. and Lysinibacillus fusiformis. Food Control. 2016;**68**:92-96

[110] Alberts JF, Gelderblom WCA, Botha A, van Zyl WH. Degradation of aflatoxin B1 by fungal laccase enzymes. International Journal of Food Microbiology. 2009;**135**:47-52

[111] Logrieco AF, Miller JD, Eskola M, Krska R, Ayalew A, Bandyopadhyay R, Battilani P, Bhatnagar D, Chulze S, De Saeger S, Li P, Perrone G, Poapolathep A, Rahayu ES, Shephard GS, Stepman F, Zhang H, Leslie JF. The Mycotox charter: Increasing awareness of, and concerted action for, minimizing mycotoxin exposure worldwide. Toxins. 2018;**10**(4):149

Section 2

Prevention and Control of Aflatoxins

Chapter 2

Effect of Harvesting Time and Drying Methods on Aflatoxin Contamination in Groundnut in Mozambique

Emmanuel Zuza Jnr, Amade Muitia,
Manuel I.V. Amane, Rick L. Brandenburg,
Andrew Emmott and Ana M. Mondjana

Additional information is available at the end of the chapter

http://dx.doi.org/10.5772/intechopen.77300

Abstract

The production and utilization of groundnut have increased tremendously across all provinces of Mozambique. However, the presence of aflatoxins has remained a critical food concern in the human diet. In this study, the effect of harvesting time and drying methods on aflatoxin contamination was examined in Northern Mozambique. A randomized complete block design in a split-split plot arrangement with four replications was used with groundnut varieties as the main plot and harvesting dates and drying methods as the subplots. Groundnut samples were analyzed for aflatoxin using the Mreader. In both locations, field observations indicated that on average, aflatoxin contamination levels were lower at physiological maturity (≤10 ppb) compared to harvesting 10 days before (≤15 ppb) and 10 days after physiological maturity (≥20 ppb). It was also observed that the two drying methods were effective in prevention of aflatoxin contamination on groundnut kernels to levels lower than 20 ppb. Aflatoxin contamination levels were significantly lower (≤12 ppb) as a result of the A-Frame than the tarpaulin method. The results of this study, therefore, have indicated that proper postharvest management of groundnuts, such as harvesting at physiological maturity and improved drying, gave lowest aflatoxin contamination levels.

Keywords: groundnut, harvesting time, aflatoxin contamination, drying methods

1. Introduction

Groundnut (*Arachis hypogaea* L.) is the third most important crop in Mozambique after maize (*Zea mays*) and cassava (*Manihot esculenta*) [1, 2]. It is a major cash crop and the main source of cooking oil for many Mozambican families [1, 3]. In terms of production, groundnut occupies the largest area among the grain legumes in the country [1, 4] with the largest concentration in Nampula, Zambezia, and Cabo Delgado provinces.

Despite its importance as food, the presence of mycotoxins, especially aflatoxins, has the potential to limit its use in both the human and livestock diet [5]. Furthermore, aflatoxin contamination of agricultural crops, such as groundnut and cereals, causes annual losses of more than US $750 million in Africa and more than US $100 million per year in USA [6]. Poor management practices by farmers and adverse climatic conditions at harvest and postharvest are some of the prompting factors for postharvest aflatoxin contamination. The timing of harvesting greatly influences mold production at harvest [7]. In [8], it is highlighted that farmers tend to delay in harvesting their crops which results in over maturity leading to mold infections and subsequent aflatoxin contamination.

Correct and proper drying of harvested groundnuts is very essential in prevention of fungal infection of the crop. Additionally, proper drying is critical for maintaining seed quality for consumption and safe storage. However, the traditional groundnut drying techniques in Mozambique involve field and bare ground drying, which rather promote fungal growth and consequent aflatoxin contamination [9]. Moreover, these are slow, time-consuming, and labor-intensive, involving lots of crop handling, and due to rains that normally persist at harvesting and drying times, it is difficult to achieve the recommended moisture content for safe storage (which is 6–8%). In addition, the crop is persistently exposed to the soil, which is a major source of contamination by fungi [10, 11].

Ideally, pods should be dried with sufficient air circulation and in the shade [10]. This is because excessive exposure to the sun can affect the quality of the seed. Two principal methods are used elsewhere in Africa, both of which can produce good quality seed with reduced levels of fungal infection [12]. These drying methods are namely Corks and A-Frame methods. However, the traditional drying techniques in Mozambique involve bare ground drying and are a major source of fungal contamination. Furthermore, some farmers do not dry groundnuts immediately after harvest, due to labor constraints needed for plucking [9]. Thus, they heap the nuts either in the field or in houses. These practices, coupled with inefficient and slow drying process under the humid conditions, enhance aflatoxin contamination greatly.

Although research on the effect of harvesting time and drying method of groundnut on aflatoxin development has received increasing consideration worldwide, in Mozambique, research on this matter is still very scarce [13]. However, there is evidence to suggest that aflatoxin contamination is a major food-safety concern in Mozambique where the environmental conditions and socio-economic problems are conducive due to poor postharvest and storage management and subsequent food spoilage and aflatoxin contamination. This is evident by the levels of certain types of cancer and the negative correlations between aflatoxin in the diet and development in children and the declining of groundnut exports from Mozambique since 1998 [13, 14].

http://dx.doi.org/10.5772/intechopen.77300

By assessing different harvesting times and different drying methods, it was hoped that the results would enhance the use of good postharvest handling practices (drying and harvesting time) that would minimize aflatoxin contamination of groundnuts at the farmer level.

2. Materials and methods

2.1. Description of the study area

The study was conducted during the 2015/2016 growing season in two locations, namely Nampula Research Station (PAN) and Mapupulo Agricultural Research Center (CIAM), located in Nampula and Cabo Delgado Provinces, respectively. Nampula Research Station (PAN) is located about 7 km east of Nampula city in Northern Mozambique (15° 09′ S, 39° 30′ E) and is elevated at 432 m above sea level. The soil type is sandy loam, and the vegetation is predominantly grassland. The average rainfall is slightly over 1000 mm which starts around November/December up to April/May, with its peak in January. The maximum temperature in the region is about 39°C and the minimum temperature is 19°C [1]. Mapupulo Agricultural Research Center (CIAM) is located about 18 km south of Montepuez town about 200 km west of Pemba the capital of the province, which lies at (13° 12′ S, 38° 53′ E) and is elevated at 476.7 m above sea level. The soils are clay loam and deep brown loam. It receives annual precipitation of 1200 mm on average from November/December to April/May, and the average temperature is between 20 and 25°C [1].

2.2. Field establishment

The study was carried out during the 2015/2016 growing season at PAN and CIAM. The test materials were evaluated using a randomized complete block design in a split-split plot arrangement with four replications. The main plot was the variety, while harvesting time and drying method were subplots. The net plots were six rows by 6-m long with one seed per planting station which were spaced at 50 cm apart, and the planting stations were spaced at 10 cm. Spanish groundnut varieties (take 90 days to mature) were used for the study, namely *ICGV-SM-99568*, *JL-24*, and *ICGV-SM-01514*. The experiments were established on 23rd and 24th December at CIAM and PAN, respectively, at the onset of the rains. No fertilizer, pesticides, or supplementary water were applied, and no seed treatment before planting was applied.

The assessment of the effect of harvesting time and drying method on aflatoxin contamination among the varieties involved dividing the net plots into three harvesting time treatments: (i) 10 days before physiological maturity indicated as H1; (ii) at physiological maturity indicated as H2, and (iii) 10 days after physiological maturity indicated as H3. The following drying treatments were imposed on the plants from each of the plots: (1) pulling and inverted windrowing of plants for 3 days, followed by further drying of the plants with the pods on constructed "A-Frames" for 4 weeks and (2) pulling and inverted windrowing of plants for 3 days, followed by stripping of the pods and further drying on interlaced tarpaulins mats for 4 weeks. The samples were later subjected to aflatoxin testing using the immune-chromatographic method mreader.

2.3. Weather data

Air temperature, relative humidity, and rainfall data were collected using weather stations on the research stations.

2.4. Determination of moisture content

The moisture content of groundnut samples was measured using the Mini GAC moisture meters. These were calibrated to ensure the accuracy. To determine the moisture content, groundnut samples were initially shelled. Later, a total of 50 g was filled in the moisture meter loader, after which the loader was emptied into the analyzer. The results were read using the display window on the moisture meters.

2.5. Aflatoxin analysis

2.5.1. Validation of the MReader

To determine the precision and recovery of the immune-chromatographic assay analysis, antigenic standards were used. For high calibration standard procedure, 100 μl of pink antigenic standard was added to 500 μl of sample buffer diluent. Then 100 μl was aliquoted in a separate vial. A reveal Q+ test strip was placed in the vial and was left to develop for 6 min. After 6 min, the strip was placed in the mreader strip holder, and the aflatoxin levels were read using the mreader. For the low calibration standard procedure, 35 ml of 65% ethanol solution was added to a 10 g control groundnut sample which was free of aflatoxins. Then, a 100 μl of the pink antigenic standard solution was added to the 30 ml extracts and mixed for 2 min. Later, a 100 μl of the mixture was added to 500 μl of the sample buffer diluent. A mixture of 100 μl was later aliquoted to a separate vial. Finally, the total aflatoxin in the sample was measured by placing the reveal Q+ test strip in the vial and was left to develop for 6 min, and aflatoxin reading was done using the mreader.

2.5.2. Sample preparation and aflatoxin determination

Aflatoxin analysis was carried out using immune-chromatographic assay Reveal Q+ mreader according to the manufacturer's recommendation. Prepared groundnut samples (500 g each) were ground finely using the Agri-Grind grinder until fine particles and homogeneity were obtained. Then, a subsample of 10 g was obtained from each of the composite samples. The subsample was aliquoting in 35 ml of 65% ethanol, and the contents were mixed gently by shaking the holding tube manually. After filtration of the blended subsample, 100 μl of the filtrate was mixed with 500 μl diluent solution in a dilution vial. After obtaining a fine mixture, a 100 μl extract of the aliquoted mixture was collected and added to a separate vial. Finally, a reveal Q+ test strip was placed in the vial containing the aliquoted mixture and was left to develop for 6 min. The test strip was later placed in the mreader holder, and the aflatoxin contamination levels of the sample were determined using the mreader based on the chromatographic characteristics of the sample in the strip. The data were statistically analyzed using GenStat Discovery 4. An independent Tukey's test was used to compare the means of the aflatoxin results. The tests for relationships were carried out using the Pearson Correlation Index, and the interpretation was performed at two-sided 95% confidence limit.

3. Results

3.1. Weather data at CIAM and PAN during 2015–2016 growing season

A summary of mean air temperature, relative humidity, and rainfall during the 2015–2016 growing season at Mapupulo Agricultural Research Center is presented in **Table 1**.

The mean daily air temperature during the pod-filling period was about 26.3°C up until H1.

Although the mean daily temperature declined to around 24.5°C by H3, the site received a total rainfall of 684.6 by H1 and 830 mm between H2 and H3, respectively, of which 50–65% fell during the pod-filling period. Additionally, there was also some postharvest rainfall during the drying period, with 37.2 mm falling between H2 and H3. The average relative humidity was between 80 and 85% during the groundnut harvesting and drying periods. However, overall there were generally high temperatures and heavy rainfall during the pod-filling till H2.

Nampula Research Station received lower rainfall during the 2015–2016 growing season compared to CIAM (**Table 2**). The site received rainfall of 299.8 mm (for only 11 days) during pod-filling, and the location experienced a mid-season drought (February).

Month	December	January	February	March	April
Average max temperature (°C)	34.1	30.5	31.4	31.9	30.8
Average min temperature (°C)	21.8	21.6	21.3	22.0	20.3
Cumulative rainfall (mm)	516.6	1300.6	568.7	800.4	859.7
Total number of rainy days	10	20	18	16	22
Relative humidity (%)	68	83	80	81	79

Table 1. Weather data during the 2015–2016 growing season at CIAM.

Month	December	January	February	March	April
Average max temperature (°C)	35.3	34.8	36.3	35.2	32
Average min temperature (°C)	33.2	29.6	32.1	32.3	29.7
Cumulative rainfall (mm)	232.9	469.6	299.8	799.1	43.9
Total number of rainy days	6	12	11	18	4
Relative humidity (%)	83	87.7	76.3	83	85

Table 2. Weather data during the 2015–2016 growing season at PAN.

However, significant higher rainfall fell during H1, while H2 and H3 experienced a prolonged end of season drought. The mean daily air temperatures during the pod-filling period at PAN were higher ranging from 30 to 35°C by H1 to H3. Additionally, the location experienced very high relative humidity ranging from 75 to 85%.

3.2. Postharvest pod handling and kernel moisture content

Moisture content of groundnut kernels greatly influences the growth of toxigenic fungi and subsequent aflatoxin contamination. The study has shown that different drying methods had different influences on the total kernel moisture losses at different experimental sites at different harvesting times. Moisture content of kernels from the A-Frame at both sites decreased from an average of 38–7%, within a 4-week period (**Figure 1**). These moisture contents were significantly different at ($P \leq 0.05$) from each other. It was observed that kernel moisture loss was rapid just after harvesting compared to the other following weeks. This was attributed to the high water activity in the seeds just after harvesting than the following weeks, which resulted into increased diffusion rate of water from the seeds to the environment through evapotranspiration and thus leading to rapid loss of water.

Significant differences ($P \leq 0.05$) were also recorded in kernel moisture loss of tarpaulin dried pods. The moisture content decreased from an average of 38–7%, within a 2-week period (**Figure 2**). It has been established that, using the tarpaulin drying method, kernel moisture loss was more rapid compared to using the A-Frame drying method. The reason behind this was that, with tarpaulin drying, pods were exposed to direct sunlight which resulted into rapid losses of kernel moisture within a short period of time, while for the A-Frame method, the kernels took a longer time to dry because the pods were facing inwards and away from the sunlight and soil and were covered by leaves. This ensured a good air circulation and slow but effective drying.

The study also revealed that the variety *JL-24* took a shorter period of time to dry compared to the other two varieties irrespective of the drying method. This could be attributed to the lower

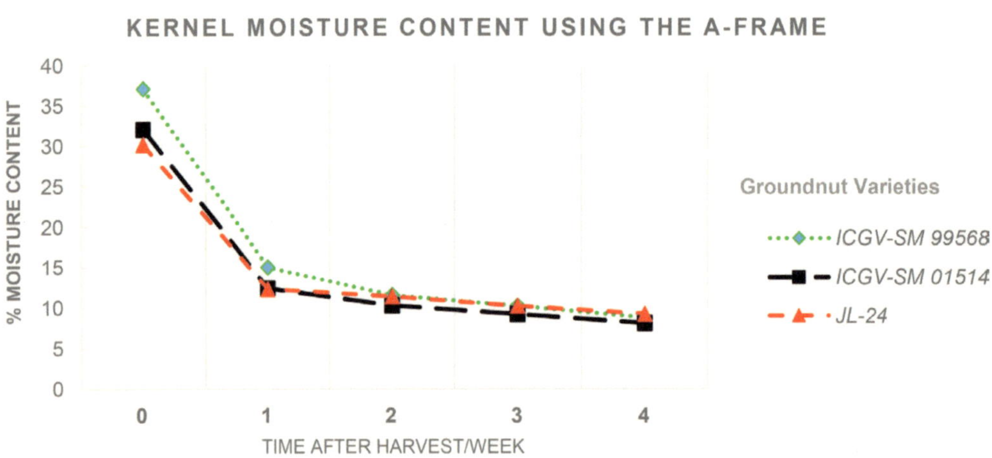

Figure 1. Kernel moisture loss when using the A-Frame.

moisture content of the variety and the thinner layer of the shell. The variety *ICGV-SM-01514* took the longest time to dry irrespective of the drying method and this could be attributed to the thicker shell of the variety which led to slower moisture loss.

3.3. Effect of harvesting time on groundnut aflatoxin contamination

Aflatoxin contamination levels among groundnut varieties at different harvesting times are presented in **Figure 3**. Significant differences ($P \leq 0.01$) were observed in the mean aflatoxin contamination levels with physiological maturity (H2) having the lowest aflatoxin contamination levels (≤10 ppb). The highest aflatoxin contamination levels were recorded when

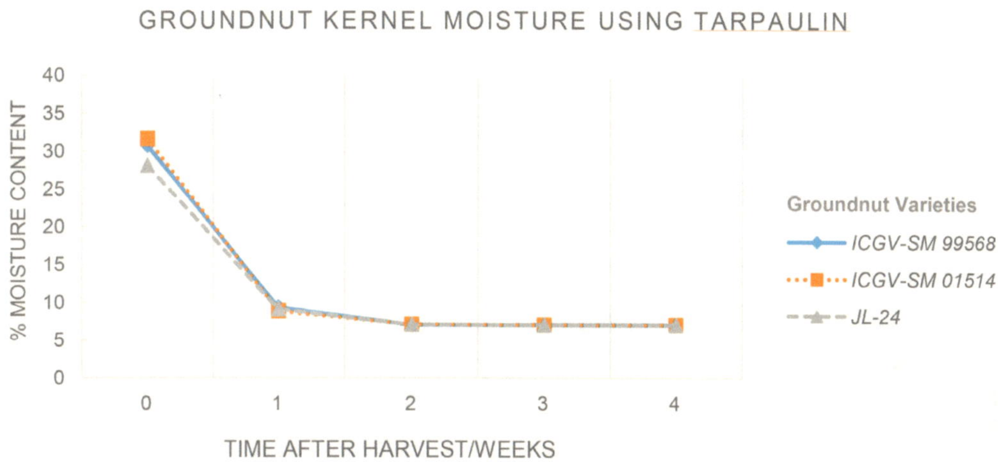

Figure 2. Kernel moisture loss when using tarpaulins.

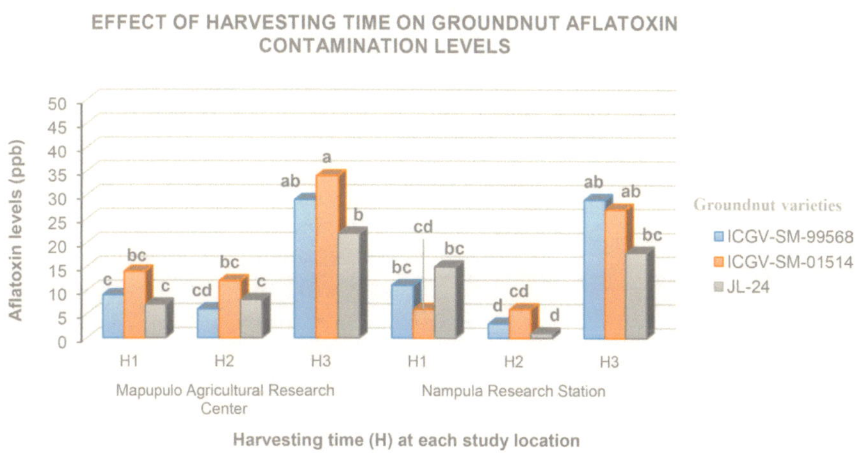

Figure 3. Aflatoxin levels in groundnuts as affected by harvesting time.

harvesting was executed 10 days after physiological maturity (H3) (≥20 ppb) compared to when harvesting was executed 10 days before physiological maturity (H1) (≤15), which had considerably lower aflatoxin levels.

The study also revealed significant differences in aflatoxin levels among the three groundnut varieties. The variety *JL-24* had the lowest mean aflatoxin contamination levels compared to the other two varieties. This could be attributed to the lower moisture content of the *JL-24* and the thin shell of the variety which led to rapid drying and minimized fungal invasion and subsequent aflatoxin contamination.

The study also revealed significant differences in aflatoxin levels among the three groundnut varieties. The variety *JL-24* had the lowest mean aflatoxin contamination levels compared to the other two varieties. This could be attributed to the lower moisture content of the *JL-24* and the thin shell of the variety which led to rapid drying and minimized fungal invasion and subsequent aflatoxin contamination. Furthermore, it was observed that at CIAM, the mean aflatoxin contamination levels of *ICGV-SM-99568* (14.5 ppb) were significantly lower compared to that of *ICGV-SM-01514* (17.9 ppb). A similar trend of results was observed at PAN; however, at this location, *ICGV-SM-01514* had the lowest mean aflatoxin contamination levels (12.3 ppb) compared to (14.3 ppb) for the variety *ICGV-SM-99568*.

3.4. Effect of drying method on groundnut aflatoxin contamination

Significant differences were observed in aflatoxin contamination levels among the groundnut varieties as a result of drying method. Lower levels of aflatoxin were recorded by the use of A-Frame compared to the tarpaulin drying method (**Figure 4**). However, except for the variety *ICGV-SM-01514* (26 ppb) at CIAM, the aflatoxin contamination levels for the groundnut varieties were lower than 20 ppb as a result of both drying methods, and thereby, showing the effectiveness of the two drying methods in prevention of aflatoxin contamination.

Significant differences in aflatoxin contamination levels were also observed among the groundnut varieties as a result of the interaction between harvesting time and drying methods

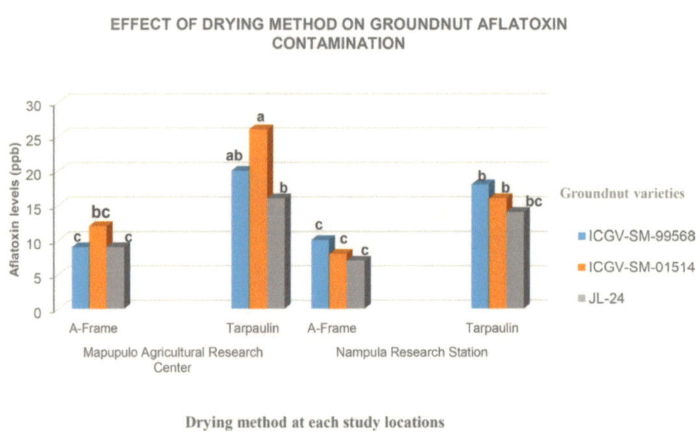

Figure 4. Effect of drying method on groundnut aflatoxin contamination.

at the two study locations (**Tables 3** and **4**). The results showed that aflatoxin contamination of the nuts started at H1 and significantly increased with delayed harvesting time (H3).

At Mapupulo Agricultural Research Center, the lowest aflatoxin contamination levels were found to be 3 and 4 ppb for the A-Frame and tarpaulin drying methods, respectively, harvested at physiological maturity. For Nampula Research Station, the lowest levels of aflatoxin contamination were found to be 2 ppb for both drying methods harvested at physiological maturity.

Higher aflatoxin levels (≥25 ppb) were recorded when harvesting was executed 10 days after physiological maturity (H3) with respect to the drying methods. In summary, it has been established that the interaction of delayed harvesting and tarpaulin drying method resulted in higher aflatoxin contamination among the groundnut varieties than the interaction of delayed harvesting and A-Frame drying method. Overall, the interaction of harvesting time and A-Frame drying method resulted into lower aflatoxin contamination levels than the interaction of harvesting time and tarpaulin drying method.

Drying method	**Variety**	**Harvest timing**		
		H1	**H2**	**H3**
A-Frame	ICGV-SM-99568	3^{c}	7^{bc}	17^{b}
	ICGV-SM-01514	10^{bc}	3^{c}	25^{a}
	JL-24	4^{c}	4^{c}	19^{ab}
Tarpaulin	ICGV-SM-99568	16^{bc}	4^{d}	40^{ab}
	ICGV-SM-01514	17^{bc}	10^{cd}	42^{a}
	JL-24	9^{cd}	13^{c}	25^{b}
Mean ± SE A-Frame 10 ± 3.77		Tarpaulin 21 ± 5.17		

Means within a column followed by the same letter are not significantly different based on Tukey's test (**P < 0.01**).

Table 3. Groundnut aflatoxin levels as affected by the interaction of harvesting time and drying method at CIAM.

Drying method	**Variety**	**Harvest timing**		
		H1	**H2**	**H3**
A-Frame	ICGV-SM-99568	3^{c}	2^{c}	27^{a}
	ICGV-SM-01514	2^{c}	2^{c}	21^{ab}
	JL-24	10^{bc}	1^{c}	12^{b}
Tarpaulin	ICGV-SM-99568	18^{b}	4^{c}	32^{a}
	ICGV-SM-01514	8^{bc}	8^{bc}	33^{a}
	JL-24	19^{b}	2^{c}	22^{ab}
Mean ± SE A-Frame 9 ± 4.03		Tarpaulin 16.5 ± 5.6		

Means within a column followed by the same letter are not significantly different based on Tukey's test (**P < 0.01**).

Table 4. Groundnut aflatoxin levels as affected by the interaction of harvesting time and drying method at PAN.

4. Discussion

A number of studies have shown that weather directly influences host susceptibility to aflatoxin contamination [15]. The differences in the intensity of aflatoxin contamination between CIAM and PAN could be attributed to the variability in intensity and duration of rainfall, temperature, and relative humidity between the two locations. In general, CIAM had significantly higher aflatoxin contamination levels compared to PAN. This was attributed to higher than normal temperatures (≥30°C) and late season rainfall which created warm, moist conditions suitable for fungal growth, and subsequent higher aflatoxin contamination levels on the kernels. These outcomes are similar to earlier accounts that wetter and more humid conditions tend to aggravate aflatoxin levels as it enhances the growth of *Aspergillus* species and production of aflatoxins in groundnuts compared to drier climatic conditions [16]. In addition, studies have shown that the optimal temperature range for production of aflatoxin is approximately 25–30°C agreeing with the current study [17].

The study also recorded higher aflatoxin contamination levels in the groundnut kernels above the recommended 20 ppb (US standards) at both CIAM and PAN. This could be as a result higher air temperatures (≥30°C) along with elevated relative humidity (≥70%) which provided optimum conditions for fungal invasion especially for the *Aspergillus* section *Flavi* and later production of aflatoxins. This was consistent with the findings of Hell and Mutegi [18] who reported that environmental conditions that favor *Aspergillus* group of fungi included high soil or air temperature (25–30°C), high relative humidity (70–85%), and drought stress.

Field observations have shown that on average, aflatoxin contamination levels were lower at physiological maturity (H2) compared to harvesting at 10 days after physiological maturity (H3). Furthermore, harvesting the crop at H1 had significantly higher aflatoxin contamination levels than harvesting at H2, with some exceptions. The high aflatoxin levels at H1 were attributed to immaturity of pods, higher pod and kernel moisture content, and adverse conditions of wet and humid weather, which provided conducive conditions for fungal invasion and consequently aflatoxin production. Additionally, most of the pods were small and shriveled, which provided direct access to the entry of microorganisms including fungi into the pods and consequently attacking the kernels and later contaminating the crop with aflatoxins. This confirmed the findings of Okello et al. [1] who reported that harvesting groundnuts too early or when the pods are immature result in high aflatoxin levels in the kernels. The findings were also consistent with the findings by Hell et al. [19] who found that aflatoxin contamination was positively correlated with wet weather during harvest (rainfall). It has also been shown that as a result of early harvesting, drying coincided with some postharvest rainfall which led into high aflatoxin contamination of the crop since there was excess moisture which provided suitable conditions for fungal growth and development and production of aflatoxins.

Harvesting 10 days after physiological maturity (H3) resulted into highest levels of aflatoxin contamination compared to H1 and H2 among the groundnut varieties in both study locations. Confirming the study findings by Mphande et al. [20] who reported that postharvest contamination with aflatoxin in groundnut increased when harvesting was executed 5 days after physiological maturity. Additionally, the study has shown that delayed harvesting resulted into higher aflatoxin contamination levels greater than the FDA/WHO regulatory levels of 20 ppb [21]. The high aflatoxin contamination levels at H3 were as a result of heavy damage of pods by insects especially termites (*Odontotermes badius* and *Odontotermes latericus*) which provided the ready entry of fungi including *Aspergillus* species and consequently aflatoxin contamination. Kombiok et al. [22] reported that insects influence the levels of aflatoxin contamination in commodities such as maize and groundnut by carrying fungal inoculum and causing damage that provide the ready entry of the fungus, and thereby increasing the chances of aflatoxin contamination. Furthermore, insects such as termites cause scarification of pods, which weakens the shells and makes them liable to crack during harvesting leading to further insect, microbial, and disease infestations [23].

High aflatoxin contamination levels at H3 could also be attributed to physical damage of pods as a result of digging using hoes. Harvesting groundnut 10 days after physiological maturity coincided with dry weather making it difficult to harvest the groundnuts by hand pulling which led to digging the nuts out of the soil using hand hoes. Similar to the effect of insect damage to pods, physical damage to pods tended to increase with delay in harvesting perhaps due to the dryness of the soil which made pulling and digging out of pods very difficult. As a result, many pods of the groundnut varieties got damaged which favored the entry and invasion of the nuts by *Aspergillus* Section *Flavi* that later produced aflatoxins as a result of respiration. These findings are concurrent with the findings of Hell et al. [18] who indicated that some factors that influence the incidence of fungal infection and subsequent toxin development include invertebrate vectors (insects), grain damage, inoculum load, substrate composition, fungal infection levels, prevalence of toxigenic strains, and microbiological interactions. Moreover, the highest levels of *A. flavus* and *A. parasiticus* infection and aflatoxin contamination are associated with seed damage caused by either insects or physical damage of pods [24].

It has also been observed that delayed harvesting coincided with high relative humidity (≥75%) and higher air/soil temperatures (30–35°C) which provided hot and moist conditions for fungal growth and subsequent aflatoxin contamination. This phenomenal confirmed the findings of Cotty and Jaime-Garcia [15] who stated that influences of delayed harvesting on aflatoxin contamination are most severe when crops are caught by higher than normal temperatures (25–30°C) and high relative humidity just prior to or during harvest (≥70%). Additionally, harvesting groundnut 10 days after physiological maturity coincided with high populations of *Aspergillus* species in the soil which led to high aflatoxin contamination.

The correct drying of harvested groundnuts is very important, as inappropriate drying can help induce fungal growth and reduce kernel quality for consumption and germination for the following season. At harvest, groundnut fruits have a higher moisture content (38–40%) and must be dried to (7–8%) to prevent growth of fungi [25]. This agrees with the current study and furthermore, the drying method greatly influences the resistance of groundnuts to fungal attack. It has been established from the results of this study that both the A-Frame and tarpaulin drying methods were effective in reducing the moisture content of groundnut to the recommended level of ≤7%, and thereby reduced the chances of heavy aflatoxin contamination on the kernels. However, the tarpaulin drying method was more rapid in reducing kernel moisture levels compared to the A-Frame dying method. This was attributed to the direct exposure of the pods to sunlight compared to the shading of pods with leaves when on the A-Frame.

Nevertheless, significant differences were observed in aflatoxin contamination levels between A-Frame and tarpaulin drying methods. Lower aflatoxin contamination levels were observed when using the A-Frame (≤10 ppb) compared to tarpaulin drying (≤20 ppb) which had to some extent higher aflatoxin contamination levels. The high aflatoxin contamination levels when using the tarpaulin method were attributed to alterations of the pod and seed coat as a result of direct exposure to sunlight which resulted into creation of microscopic poles and cracks that provided the ready entry of fungi and later aflatoxin production. The advantage of the A-Frame drying method over tarpaulin drying was that it prevented direct exposure of the pods to sunlight and provided increased air circulation as a result of the pods being on a raised platform which led to efficient and effective drying resulting into lower fungal invasion. This confirmed the findings that if drying is too rapid, there are alterations in the seed coat that favor fungal infection [26].

High aflatoxin contamination levels with the tarpaulin drying method could also be as a result of weather conditions. Postharvest abrupt rainfall during the drying period resulted into wetting of pods and prevented drying of the pods to the open sun on some days when it rained all day which resulted into creation of moist conditions conducive for aflatoxin production by the fungi. This was not the case with the A-frame since the pods were covered with leaves and thereby preventing water from reaching the pods and ensuring exposure to air circulation all the time. One of the disadvantages of drying groundnuts on tarpaulins is the time and effort required to gather the pods together and cover them during rain showers and respreading the pods as soon as possible in order to continue drying; this is difficult and the adverse moist conditions as a result of rain provided optimum conditions for fungal invasion and aflatoxin production.

However, in general, it has been observed that both the A-frame and the tarpaulin drying methods were effective in prevention of aflatoxin contamination of the groundnut crop than would traditional methods of drying which involve field and bare ground drying. Furthermore, the A-frame and tarpaulin drying methods ensured that the groundnut crop attained the recommended moisture content (≤7%) and ensured that the crop was not in direct contact with the soil, thereby preventing easy access of fungi to the pods and thus ensuring minimum fungal invasion.

5. Conclusions and recommendations

The results of the assessment of different harvesting times and different drying methods are rather obvious (and confirm previous studies), namely (a) harvesting 10 days after physiological maturity (H3) results into the highest levels of aflatoxin, (b) harvesting groundnuts too early or when the pods are immature results in high aflatoxin levels in the kernels, (c) physical damage of pods as a result of digging using hoes (there is not much of an alternative when harvesting during dry weather), (d) insects influence the levels of aflatoxin contamination, and (e) A-frame and the tarpaulin drying are more effective in reducing aflatoxin contamination of groundnuts. However, the implementation of those good postharvest handling practices (drying and harvesting time) requires a close monitoring at the farmer level.

http://dx.doi.org/10.5772/intechopen.77300

It may be interesting to research the constraints by adopting such practices (when farmers are knowledgeable about the problem). Besides, it is difficult to avoid in the studied areas of Mozambique the ideal situation of an optimal temperature range for production of aflatoxin (between 25 and 30°C). Wet and more humid conditions quite evidently aggravate aflatoxin levels. Scenarios may be useful to better understand the necessary trade-offs to be made by the farmer to optimize harvesting times and drying method depending on the local context (availability of tarpaulin, A-frames, or Mandela Cork dying methods) and weather forecasts. An assessment of the conditions under which [waiting for] physiological maturity is difficult to respect would have been useful and the reasons why damage to the pods cannot be avoided.

Acknowledgements

This publication was made possible through the support provided by the Office of Agriculture, Research and Policy, Bureau of Food Security, U.S. Agency for International Development, under the terms of Award No. AID-ECG-A-00-07-0001 to the University of Georgia as management entity for the U.S. Feed the Future Innovation Lab on Peanut Productivity and Mycotoxin Control. The authors would also like to acknowledge the support provided by the Institute of Agricultural Investigation of Mozambique and Eduardo Mondlane University. Special thanks to Limbikani Matumba and Wezi Mhango for provision of useful insights during the research period.

Conflict of interest

The opinions expressed herein are those of the author(s) and do not necessarily reflect the views of the U.S. Agency for International Development.

Author details

Emmanuel Zuza Jnr[1*], Amade Muitia[2], Manuel I.V. Amane[3], Rick L. Brandenburg[4], Andrew Emmott[5] and Ana M. Mondjana[1]

*Address all correspondence to: manzyzuzajnr@gmail.com

1 Department of Crop Protection, Faculty of Agriculture and Forestry Engineering, Eduardo Mondlane University, Maputo, Mozambique

2 Nampula Research Station, Nampula, Mozambique

3 Institute of Agriculture Investigation of Mozambique, Maputo, Mozambique

4 Department of Entomology, Center for Turfgrass Environmental Research and Education, North Carolina State University, Raleigh, North Carolina, United States of America

5 Nut Cellars, Bedford, United Kingdom

References

[1] Muitia A. Farmer perceptions and genetic studies of rosette disease in groundnut (*Arachis hypogaea* L.) in northern Mozambique [PhD thesis]. KwaZulu-Natal: African Centre for Crop Improvement; 2013

[2] Walker T, Pitoro R, Tomo A, Sitoe I, Salencia C, Mahanzule R, et al. Priority Setting for Public-Sector Agricultural Research in Mozambique with the National Agricultural Survey Data. Maputo, Mozambique: Ministry of Agriculture of Mozambique; 2006

[3] IIAM, Muitia A. Combination of root-knot nematodes (*Meloidogyne* spp.) resistance and edible seed quality for peanut (*Arachis hypogaea* L.) production in Mozambique and in the U.S. Lubbock, Texas [MSc thesis]. Texas Tech University; 2005

[4] Arias FJ, Libombo ML. Groundnut evaluation in Mozambique: Preliminary results from the 1993/94 season in Maputo Province. In: Ndunguru BJ et al., editors. Sustainable Groundnut Production in South and Eastern Africa. Swaziland, Mbabane: International Crops Research Institute for the Semi-Arid Tropics; 1994

[5] Rahmianna AA, Taufiq A, Yusnawan E. Effect of harvest timing and postharvest storage conditions on aflatoxin contamination in groundnuts harvested from the Wonogiri regency in Indonesia. SAT eJournal. 2005;**5**:1-3

[6] Kamika I, Takoy LL. Natural occurrence of aflatoxin B1 in peanut collected from Kinshasa, Democratic Republic of Congo. Food Control. 2011;**22**:1760-1764

[7] Guo BZ, Sobolev V, Holbrook CC, Lynch RE. Impact of phytoalexins and lesser cornstalk borer damage on resistance to aflatoxin contamination. Phytopathology. 2013;**93**:S31

[8] Wright G, Rachaputi N, Chauhan Y, Robson A. Increasing productivity and quality of peanuts using novel crop modeling and remote sensing technologies. In: International Peanut Conference. Bangkok, Thailand: Kasetsart University; 2005. pp. 9-12

[9] Jeffrey EE. Groundnut Grower's Guide for Mozambique: Production, Harvesting and Post-Harvest Handling. Mozambique: CNFA; 2011

[10] Okello KD, Archileo NK, Jenipher B, Moreen W, Herbert KO. Management of Aflatoxins in Groundnuts; A Manual for Farmers, Processors, Traders and Consumers in Uganda. Entebbe: National Agricultural Research Organisation; 2010

[11] Kaaya AN, Kyamuhangire W, Kyamanywa S. Factors affecting aflatoxin contamination of harvested maize in the three agroecological zones of Uganda. Journal of Applied Sciences. 2007;**6**:2401-2407

[12] AICC (African Institute of Corporate Citizenship). Harmonized Groundnut Production Manual for Malawi. Lilongwe: Business Support Technology; 2014

[13] Almeida Z, Nicolas R. Mitigation of Aflatoxin in Maize and Groundnuts in Mozambique. Mozambique: USAID; 2013

[14] FAO-STAT. Country Profile: Mozambique. Groundnut Production Trends. Food and Agricultural Organization of the United Nations; 2015

[15] Cotty PJ, Jaime-Gracia R. Influence of climate on aflatoxin producing fungi and aflatoxin contamination. International Journal of Food Microbiology. 2007;**119**:109-115

[16] Menza NC, Muturi WM, Kamau ML. Incidence, types and levels of aflatoxin in different peanuts varieties produced in Busia and Kisii Central Districts, Kenya. Open Journal of Medical Microbiology. 2015;**5**:209-221

[17] Widstrom NW, Butron A, Guo BZ, Wilson DM, Snook ME, Cleveland TE, et al. Control of pre-harvest aflatoxin contamination in maize by pyramiding QTL involved in resistance to ear-feeding insects and invasion by Aspergillus spp. European Journal of Agronomy. 2003;**19**(4):563-572

[18] Hell K, Mutegi C. Aflatoxin control and prevention strategies in key crops of sub-Saharan Africa. African Journal of Microbiology Research. 2011;**5**(5):459-466

[19] Hell K, Cardwell KF, Poehling HM. Relationship between management practices, fungal infection and aflatoxin for stored groundnuts in Benin. Journal of Phytopathology. 2003;**151**:690-698

[20] Mphande FA, Siame BA, Taylor JE. Fungi, aflatoxins and cyclopiazonic acid associated with peanut retailing in Botswana. Journal of Food Protection. 2004;**67**:96-102

[21] Dowd PF. Insect management to facilitate preharvest mycotoxin management. Journal of Toxicology - Toxin Reviews. 2003;**22**(2-3):327-350

[22] Kombiok JM, Buah1 SSJ, Dzomeku IK, Abdulai H. Sources of pod yield losses in groundnut in the northern Savanna zone of Ghana. West Africa Journal of Applied Ecology. 2012;**20**(2):53-63

[23] Horn BW. Colonization of wounded peanut seeds by soil fungi: Selectivity for species from *Aspergillus* section Flavi. Mycologia. 2005;**97**(1):202-217

[24] Waliyar F, Osiru M, Ntare BR, Vijay Krishna Kumar K, Sudini H, Traore A, et al. Post-harvest management of aflatoxin contamination in groundnut. World Mycotoxin Journal. 2015;**8**(2):245-252

[25] Fernandez EM, Rosolem CM, Maringoni AC, Oliveira DMT. Fungus incidence on peanut grains as affected by drying method and Ca nutrition. Field Crops Research. 1997;**52**:9-15

[26] Nautiyal PC. Groundnut Post Harvest Operations, Post Harvest Compendium. Rome: Food and Agriculture Organization of the United Nations; 2002

Chapter 3

Preharvest Management Strategies and Their Impact on Mycotoxigenic Fungi and Associated Mycotoxins

Lindy J. Rose, Sheila Okoth, Bradley C. Flett,
Belinda Janse van Rensburg and Altus Viljoen

Additional information is available at the end of the chapter

http://dx.doi.org/10.5772/intechopen.76808

Abstract

Mycotoxigenic fungi that contaminate grain crops can lead to reduced grain quality, crop yield reduction and mycotoxicosis among humans and livestock. Preharvest management of fungi and mycotoxin contamination is considered among the most important mitigating strategies. Approaches include the breeding of resistant cultivars, use of microorganisms chemical control, production practises and the management of plant stressors. Resistant plants provide an effective and environmentally sound strategy to control mycotoxigenic fungi and mycotoxins; and have been documented. Their incorporation into commercial cultivars is, however, slow and complex. Therefore, emphasis should be placed on determining the resistance of cultivars and landraces currently used by producers. Chemical control has been successfully used for wheat; yet little to no research has been done on other important crops. Biological control strategies have focussed on *Aspergillus flavus* that produces aflatoxins and infects commercially important crops like maize and groundnuts. Commercial biological control products have been developed and field-tested in several African countries with promising results. The impacts of production practises are unclear under variable environmental conditions; but subsequent disease manifestation and mycotoxin contamination can be reduced. Each preharvest approaches contribute to managing mycotoxigenic fungi and their mycotoxins but integrating approaches may provide more effective management of fungal and mycotoxin contamination in crops.

Keywords: preharvest management, mycotoxins, tolerance, cereals, cultural practices

1. Introduction

The contamination of food and feed crops with mycotoxigenic fungi is a persistent problem contributing to food safety and security worldwide. The infection of crops by these fungal pathogens affects crop yield and quality but of greater concern are the secondary metabolites they produce, collectively known as mycotoxins. Ingestion of mycotoxin-contaminated products has been associated with a wide range of noxious effects on humans and livestock. The major food and feed crops affected by mycotoxigenic fungi and mycotoxins include rice, maize, wheat, soybean, sorghum and groundnut, although several other crops are also affected. The association of these crops with mycotoxigenic fungi is ubiquitous, and crops are affected wherever they are produced. Three major groups of mycotoxigenic fungi are associated with mycotoxin contamination namely *Aspergillus*, *Fusarium* and *Penicillium*. They each produce a number of mycotoxins, but six mycotoxins have been studied extensively and are considered among the most important and they include the aflatoxins (AF), fumonisins (FUM), trichothecenes (TCT), zearalenone (ZEA), ochratoxin (OT) and patulin (PAT). Mycotoxin contamination levels in food and feed crops have therefore elicited numerous countries to institute regulations regarding the maximum permissible levels of these mycotoxins in unprocessed and processed products.

More than 100 countries have established mycotoxin regulations, including 15 African countries [1–3]. The European Union and United States Food and Drug Administration established maximum allowable levels for certain food contaminants, including mycotoxins, with the aim to reduce their presence in foodstuffs to the lowest levels reasonably achievable by means of good manufacturing or agricultural practices [4]. Most of the countries have mycotoxin regulations for at least AFB1, produced predominantly by *Aspergillus* spp., to aid in minimising food safety concerns. Although fewer countries regulate *Fusarium* mycotoxins, a marked increase in the regulation of this mycotoxin has been observed recently. These regulations have globally significant implications for the importation and exportation of products. Regulatory infrastructure, however, does not enable inspection and enforcement [5], making the regulatory control of mycotoxins in Africa largely ineffective [6].

The management of mycotoxigenic fungi and their subsequent mycotoxins is therefore vital towards ensuring sustainable, safe food and feed production. Integrated management practises that reduce the incidence of mycotoxigenic fungi as well as the management of abiotic factors that contribute to mycotoxin contamination are required before and following harvest. However, preharvest management is considered the most important in limiting the overall contamination of crops. Therefore, the use of tolerant varieties is deemed the most proficient and environmentally sound approach to manage fungi and their toxins. In addition, several other management approaches such as optimal plant production, cultural practises, chemical control and the management of mycotoxigenic fungi by atoxigenic strains or bacteria could further reduce fungal incidence and subsequent mycotoxin contamination.

2. Management of mycotoxigenic fungi and their mycotoxins

Managing mycotoxigenic fungi and their mycotoxins in crop plants requires a proper understanding of the biology, epidemiology and genetics/genomics of the fungus and host plant. Major crops vary significantly in susceptibility to mycotoxigenic fungi and subsequent mycotoxin contamination. Maize is widely considered to be among the most susceptible of major crops to mycotoxins, while rice is considered among the least susceptible crop [7–9].

2.1. Tolerance to mycotoxigenic fungi

Crops with resistance to numerous mycotoxigenic fungi have been documented [10–12], but none of these are immune. Resistance to mycotoxigenic fungi therefore appears to be quantitative rather than qualitative. Breeding programmes at both public and private institutions are initiating and expanding their efforts to develop disease-resistant inbred and hybrid materials [13]. A number of international institutions such as the International Maize and Wheat Improvement Centre (CIMMYT) and the International Institute of Tropical Agriculture (IITA) in African countries including Kenya and Nigeria have established breeding programmes with the primary focus on producing inbred lines with improved resistance to *A. flavus* and AF. The development of tolerant cultivars, however, has been slow due to the polygenic, quantitative nature of resistance to mycotoxigenic fungi [14–17], the unavailability of immune germplasm [11, 15] and the effect of the environment on disease development and mycotoxin production [18–20]. The development of tolerant varieties, therefore, may be a long (8–10 years) and costly process that needs to be conducted as effectively as possible. Little to no commercial plant crop, completely resistant to mycotoxigenic fungi and mycotoxins, has been produced by conventional breeding, with the exception of wheat [21–23].

2.2. Conventional breeding strategies

Diallel analysis to determine the general combinability (GC) and specific combinability (SC) of resistant genotypes has been reported for *Aspergillus* and *Fusarium*, mostly performed on maize [24–27] and wheat [28–30]. The response of an inbred line to *F. verticillioides* and FUM, and the corresponding GC in hybrids, was significantly correlated. This indicates that an efficient way to improve resistance to *F. verticillioides* and FUM in maize hybrids, specifically, is to first evaluate and select resistant inbred lines that can be used to develop resistant hybrids [24]. This was also demonstrated for breeding resistance to Fusarium head blight (FHB) of wheat [30]. Maize hybrid performance for resistance to *F. graminearum* could, however, not be predicted based on the GC of inbred line parents [27]. Therefore, this relationship needs to be determined for each crop and fungal pathogen, respectively.

Inbred lines with resistance to aflatoxin contamination were evaluated for GCA and SCA for resistance to fumonisin accumulation, and two lines with resistance to FUM and AF were registered [25]. That research demonstrated the ability to breed resistance to multiple mycotoxigenic fungi and/or their mycotoxins. Furthermore, improved resistance to *F. verticillioides* and FUM in inbred lines derived from cross-pollination of resistant and elite maize lines has been demonstrated [31]. The subsequent hybrids produced from the crossing of improved lines with elite lines, however, did not demonstrate an improved activity against Fusarium ear rot (FER) and FUM accumulation, although some improved lines performed well as an inbred line and as a component of a hybrid [31]. To date, little to no research is reported on the development of tolerant varieties using recurrent selection breeding methods. Considering that resistance to mycotoxigenic fungi is polygenic and quantitative, recurrent selection presents a feasible breeding strategy; however, time and cost involved in this breeding strategy may be strong deterrent factors.

Quantitative trait loci (QTL) associated with resistance to mycotoxigenic fungi has been mapped in maize and wheat and can be used for marker-assisted selection [15, 16, 32–36]. Some QTLs, however, displayed pleiotropic effects, sometimes resulting in resistance to both traits [15, 32, 37]. QTL analyses have also demonstrated pleiotropic effects for resistance to other mycotoxigenic fungi and/or their associated mycotoxins. In QTL studies involving multiple ear rot pathogens, maize resistant to FER and FUM accumulation was also resistant to *F. graminearum* and/or *A. flavus*, with common loci for ear rots and FUM, respectively [15, 37, 38]. Research revealed that some of the genes involved in resistance to FER and Aspergillus ear rot (AER) of maize caused by *A. flavus*, as well as their associated mycotoxins (FUM and AF, respectively), were identical or genetically linked [38]. These studies highlighted common genes and/or resistance mechanisms to multiple mycotoxigenic fungi, demonstrating the potential for breeding resistance to one type of mycotoxigenic fungus, and its mycotoxin may lead to similar responses among other mycotoxigenic fungi and associated mycotoxin. The value of marker-assisted selection for improving Fusarium head blight resistance in wheat has been confirmed by numerous researchers and success stories from breeding programmes implementing MAS [39–47].

2.3. Unconventional breeding strategies

2.3.1. Genetic modification

Genetically modified crops are plants of which the DNA has been altered through the introduction of a foreign gene to express a trait not inherent to the modified plant. Three transgene-mediated strategies have been proposed for the management of mycotoxigenic fungi and mycotoxins in maize [48]. These include (1) the reduction of fungal infection, (2) the degradation of mycotoxins and (3) interfering with the mycotoxin biosynthetic pathway. To reduce infection by the fungus, the incorporation of antifungal and/or resistance genes, as well as the overexpression of defence-related genes, is required. Catabolic enzymes from microbes have been used to detoxify certain mycotoxins both *in vitro* and *in situ*, before they accumulate in the plant [49–51]. Fumonisin esterase and amine oxidase genes encoding FUM-degrading enzymes have been identified in *Exophiala spinifera* de Hoog and Hasse [48]. None of these genes have, however, been successfully introduced into maize. Maize plants have, however, been genetically engineered to interfere with the biosynthesis of AF and TCT [52, 53]. The best-known example of using genetically modified maize for reducing FER and FUM contamination of grain is Bt maize [54, 55]. This is due to the close association between kernel damage by insects and infection by *F. verticillioides* [56]. Bt maize plants that prevent insect damage, therefore, also reduce FUM contamination of maize grain. Genetically modified maize is not authorised in all countries and, consequently, conventional breeding efforts are still commonly used.

2.3.2. Mutation breeding

Exposure of seeds or other heritable materials to chemicals or radiation with the purpose to induce DNA changes (mutations) is known as mutation breeding. Nuclear technology for crop improvement makes use of ionising radiation, which causes induced mutations with a high mutation frequency in plants [57]. These mutations might be beneficial and alter physiological characters of plants, including plant height, ear height and improved root architecture [58, 59]. The radiation of seeds may also cause genetic variability that enables breeders to select new genotypes with improved grain yield and quality [60]. Mutation breeding has been successfully used to generate genetic variation in cereal crops, including maize, for a number of aspects including enhanced yield and productivity, altered ear length, drought tolerance and enhanced stem structure [61–63]. It can thus potentially provide an attractive means for generating tolerance to mycotoxigenic fungi and their mycotoxins.

2.4. Host-plant resistance

The planting of disease-resistant plants is an effective, affordable and environmentally sound strategy to control ear rot diseases and mycotoxin accumulation [64]. Commercial hybrids differ in their ability to accumulate mycotoxins [64], while hybrids grown outside of their adapted range are more susceptible to mycotoxins than those grown within their adapted range [18]. Determining host-plant resistance to mycotoxigenic fungi and mycotoxin accumulation is a fundamental step towards developing commercially tolerant plant varieties. Several factors require careful consideration when screening materials for resistance to mycotoxigenic fungi and their mycotoxins. Inoculation technique significantly contributes to the efficacy of the screening protocol and should, therefore, be appropriate, produce consistent results and consider the disease cycle of the pathogen. Numerous studies relating to different crops report on the importance of screening for resistance under variable environmental conditions since genotype by environment interactions (GEI) plays such a vital role in disease development and mycotoxin contamination. Furthermore, GEI and stability indicators provide for the selection of material tolerant across a broad range of environments or alternatively exhibiting tolerance in specific environments.

Various countries have reported on the tolerance levels of maize and wheat cultivars to mycotoxigenic fungi and associated mycotoxins [65–67]. However, focus has been placed on the characterisation of inbred lines for the identification of appropriate breeding material towards resistance to mycotoxigenic fungi and their toxins [68–74]. Genetically modified maize, expressing *Bacillus thuringiensis* genes (BT maize), has been found to accumulate less FUM than its non-modified isolines [54].

2.5. Cultural preharvest management strategies

2.5.1. Planting recommendations

Adhering to planting dates and planting plants at lower or optimal densities reduces mycotoxin accumulation during production [75–77]. Plants should be planted at recommended row widths and densities to specifically reduce water stress [78] and ensure optimal nutrient availability. Maize ears should be harvested from the field as soon as possible because favourable conditions for ear rot and/or mycotoxin accumulation may occur if harvest is delayed, thus leading to elevated mycotoxin levels [79, 80].

2.5.2. Crop rotation

The primary objective of cultural control of mycotoxigenic fungi is to minimise factors that result in plant stress. Inoculum build-up on plant residues can be reduced by crop rotation practices, such as the rotation of maize with non-host crops [75, 81, 82]. Crop rotation with legumes, brassicas and potato could also significantly reduce *F. graminearum* contamination levels [83].

2.5.3. Tillage practises

Field preparation and cultivation practices play a central role in the management of *Fusarium* diseases and associated mycotoxins [84]. The burial of plant residues from a previous planting season by deep ploughing can reduce the primary inoculum that causes infections [85]. This is especially important when crops are affected by the same *Fusarium* species, such as *F. graminearum* on maize, wheat and sorghum grown in rotation [4]. While minimum tillage has significantly decreased stalk rot and increased grain yield of sorghum in South Africa [86], it has also increased inoculum build-up of mycotoxigenic fungi in maize cropping systems [84]. Alternate tillage practices, however, have had little effect on the incidence of FER in maize [87, 88].

2.5.4. Managing plant stressors

Limiting plant stress to increase plant vigour by adhering to optimum plant dates, preventing drought stress and the optimal use of fertilisers have reduced *Fusarium* infection in a number of grain crops [76, 89–91]. However, maize cultivated by means of organic agriculture does not accumulate less FUM than maize cultivated conventionally [92, 93]. Extended periods of heat and drought stress that lead to increased FUM levels could be managed with proper irrigation schedules [77, 94]. Managing plant stress conditions is also important as this is considered key in the symptomless endophytic relationship converting to a disease- and/or mycotoxin-producing interaction [95].

2.5.5. Chemical control

Fungicides have been shown to significantly reduce FHB and DON contamination of wheat grain. Triazole fungicides such as metconazole and tebuconazole have been shown to control FHB and DON contamination in wheat [96]. However, fungicides are neither effective in reducing *F. verticillioides* infection/FUM accumulation, nor *A. flavus* infection/AF accumulation in maize [97]. This may be due to the husks that cover maize kernels. FUM were, however, reduced by 95% *in vitro* when four fungicides and a biocontrol bacterium (Serenade, *B. subtilis*) were evaluated for the control of *F. verticillioides* and *A. flavus* [98]. No registered fungicides are available for the control of either *F. verticillioides* or *A. flavus* in any African country [98]. The use of insecticides can prevent insect wounds that contribute to fungal infection and mycotoxin accumulation in maize kernels [91].

Reduced FHB severity and mycotoxin contamination of wheat under field conditions using tannic acid and the botanicals, Chinese galls and buckthorn, have been shown [100]. These researchers also reported disease and mycotoxin reduction efficacy close to that observed with a synthetic fungicide, thereby demonstrating the potential use of natural compounds in managing mycotoxigenic fungi and their toxins. Furthermore, several studies report on a reduced fungal growth and mycotoxin contamination for *Aspergillus* and *Fusarium* using natural oils and phenolic compounds *in vitro*; however, the commercial value of such products has not been explored and may not be feasible [101, 102].

2.5.6. Managing mycotoxigenic fungi with other microorganisms

The use of biological control agents to manage mycotoxigenic fungi has been reported. Atoxigenic *F. verticillioides* strains competitively excluded FUM-producing strains and prevented them from producing FUM [103]. When these strains were applied by themselves through the silk channel, however, they resulted in high levels of FER. The effective control of toxigenic *F. verticillioides* and *F. proliferatum* by non-toxigenic *Fusarium* species in maize residues has also been observed [104]. Most success, however, has been achieved with the use of atoxigenic strains of *A. flavus* to control toxigenic *A. flavus* and *A. parasiticus*. When introduced into the soil, these atoxigenic strains reduced AF contamination of peanuts in the USA by 74.3–99.9% [105]. Atoxigenic *A. flavus* strains are now widely used to control AF in maize in several African countries (www.aflatoxinpartnership.org). Endophytic bacteria have been reported to control FUM-producing fungi by competitive exclusion [106], while *Trichoderma* strains controlled them through competition for nutrients and space, fungistasis, antibiosis, rhizosphere modification, mycoparasitism, biofertilisation and the stimulation of plant-defence mechanisms [107].

2.5.7. Prediction systems

An epidemic can be described as a 'change in disease intensity in a host population over time and space' [108]. Mathematical modelling of crop disease is a rapidly expanding discipline within plant pathology [109] with the first models developed by Van der Plank [110, 111]. In epidemiology, modelling aims to understand the main determinants of epidemic development in order to address disease management in a sustainable and efficient manner. It can, therefore, serve as an instrument to monitor and assess the risk of mycotoxin contamination in crops that would drive agronomic decisions during cultivation, in order to enhance management strategies [112].

Most research regarding disease forecasting of mycotoxigenic fungi has focussed on FHB of wheat. This disease is considered well suited for risk assessment modelling because of the severity of epidemics, compound losses resulting from mycotoxin contamination and relatively narrow time periods of pathogen sporulation, inoculum dispersal and host infection [113]. This can be seen from the online forecasting model FusaProg [114], which is a threshold-based tool to control *F. graminearum* with the optimised timing of fungicide applications and forecasts of DON content during flowering. DONCast is a prediction model from Canada that has been extensively validated and commercialised for wheat [112], while an adaption of this model has been proposed for maize. This model predicts the variation in mycotoxin levels associated with the year and agronomic effects from simple linear models using wheat samples from farmers. The DONCast model accounts for up to 80% of the variation in DON and is commercially employed for the past 10 years.

Field-based models to predict FUM B1 contamination in maize grain have been elusive, most probably due to the complexity of interactions between numerous abiotic and biotic disease factors [115]. The concentration and severity of FUM produced by *Fusarium* spp. varies with meteorological conditions, genotype and location [19]. In general, favourable conditions for *F. verticillioides* infection include high temperatures [56], drought stress [56, 116] and insect damage stress [56]. A mathematical simulation of the growth of *F. graminearum* and *F. verticillioides* in maize ears was developed; however, the model only simulates fungal growth and not mycotoxin accumulation [117]. A preliminary model developed in the Philippines and Argentina identified four weather periods near silking as critical to FUM accumulation at harvest [19]. This model accounted for 82% of the variability of total FUM across all locations in 2 years of study, but did not consider meteorological conditions during grain maturation when FUM are synthesised.

A risk assessment model (FUMAgrain) developed for FUM contamination of maize grain in Italy gives an initial risk alert at the end of flowering based on meteorological conditions [118]. A second alert follows at kernel maturation following assessments of grain moisture, European corn borer damage and FUM synthesis risk. FUMAgrain could simulate FUM synthesis in maize accounting for 70% of the variation for calibration and 71% for validation. The importance of meteorological conditions at flowering and the growth of *F. verticillioides* and FUM synthesis during grain maturation was emphasised as the most important factors contributing to FUM contamination [118]. Another model consistently identified mean maximum temperature and minimum humidity as driving variables in the colonisation of maize kernels by fumonisin-producing *Fusarium* spp [99]. Furthermore, *Fusarium* colonisation of grain and fumonisins were related to prevailing weather conditions during early post-flowering and dough stage of grain development, respectively [99]. A prediction model using variables such as cultivar, climate, management practice, soil type, phenological stages of the host plant and pathogen variation would be advantages in identifying areas with potentially dangerous levels of fungal contamination and associated mycotoxin production, enabling them to implement mycotoxin management strategies.

3. Conclusion

Food and feed crops are consistently threatened by mycotoxigenic fungi and compound their infection by depositing toxic metabolites, including mycotoxins. Preharvest management of mycotoxin contamination is vital to maintaining contamination levels below economically feasible and legislated thresholds. Planting genotypes with enhanced host resistance is considered the most practical, affordable and environmentally sound method of controlling mycotoxigenic fungi and their mycotoxins. However, integrating resistant varieties with good agricultural practises such as crop rotation, chemical/biological control and other strategies that optimise plant production by minimising stressors may further reduce the risks associated with mycotoxin contamination. Resistance to mycotoxigenic fungi exists and has been identified in appropriate breeding materials but such resistance needs to be introduced in high-yielding and locally adapted hybrids. To date, conventional breeding has not been able to introgress disease and/or mycotoxin resistance into important staple crops like maize. Therefore, further research is required into factors with a greater efficacy to reduce mycotoxigenic fungi and mycotoxins preharvest as resistant varieties are being developed.

Acknowledgements

The South African Maize Trust and the National Research Foundation (NRF) of South Africa (Thuthuka; South Africa—Kenya Research Partnership Programme Bilateral); the MAIZE Competitive Grants Initiative, International Maize and Wheat Improvement Centre (CIMMYT), and CGIAR, the National Commission for Science, Technology and Innovation (NACOSTI) of Kenya; the Agricultural Research Council of South Africa are all acknowledged for funding.

Conflict of interest

The authors declare no conflict of interest.

Author details

Lindy J. Rose[1]*, Sheila Okoth[2], Bradley C. Flett[3], Belinda Janse van Rensburg[3] and Altus Viljoen[1]

*Address all correspondence to: lindym@sun.ac.za

1 Stellenbosch University, Stellenbosch, South Africa

2 University of Nairobi, Nairobi, Kenya

3 Agricultural Research Council, Potchefstroom, South Africa

References

[1] Van Egmond HP. Worldwide regulations for mycotoxins. Advances in Experimental Medicine and Biology. 2002;**504**:257-269

[2] Barug D, Van Egmond H, Lopez-Garcia R, Van Osenbruggen T, Visconti A. In: Meeting the Mycotoxins Menace. The Netherlands: Wageningen Academic Publishers; 2003

[3] Fellinger A. Worldwide mycotoxin regulations and analytical challenges. In: World Grain Summit: Foods and Beverages; 17-20 September. Vol. 2006. California, USA: San Francisco; 2006

[4] Beukes I, Rose LJ, Shephard GS, Flett BC, Viljoen A. Mycotoxigenic *Fusarium* species associated with grain crops in South Africa—A review. South African Journal of Science. 2017;**773**:3. DOI: 10.17159/sajs.2017/20160121

[5] Warburton ML, Williams WP. Aflatoxin resistance in maize: What have we learned lately? Advances in Botany. 2014;**2014**:10. Article ID: 352831. https://doi.org/10.1155/2014/352831

[6] Strosnider H, Azziz-Baumgartner E, Banziger M, Bhat RV, Breiman R, Brune MN, DeCock K, Dilley A, Groopman J, Hell K, Henry SH, Jeffers D, Jolly C, Jolly P, Kibata GN, Lewis L, Liu X, Luber G, McCoy L, Mensah P, Miraglia M, Misore A, Njapau H, Ong CN, Onsongo MT, Page SW, Park D, Patel M, Phillips T, Pineiro M, Pronczuk J, Rogers HS, Rubin C, Sabino M, Schaafsma A, Shephard G, Stroka J, Wild C, Williams JT, Wilson D. Health strategies for reducing Aflatoxin exposure in developing countries. A Workgroup Report. Environmental Health Perspectives. 2006;**12**:1898-1903

[7] Abbas HK, Cartwright RD, Windham GL, Xie W, Shier WT, Mirocha CJ. The presence of mycotoxins and fungi in rice and corn in the southern United States. Bulletin of the Institute for Comprehensive Agricultural Science, Kinki University. 2000;**8**:21-34

[8] Abbas HK, Williams WP, Windham GL, Pringle Jr JC, Xie W, Shier WT. Aflatoxin and Fumonisin contamination of commercial corn (*Zea mays*) hybrids in Mississippi. Journal of Agricultural Food Chemistry. 2002;**50**:5246-5254

[9] Reddy KRN, Abbas HK, Abel CA, Muralidharan K. Mycotoxigenic fungi, mycotoxins, and management of rice grains. Toxin Reviews. 2008;**27**:287-317

[10] Nankam C, Pataky KK. Resistance to kernel infection by *Fusarium moniliforme* in the sweet corn inbred IL 125b. Plant Disease. 1996;**80**:593-598

[11] Clements MJ, Maragos CM, Pataky JK, White DG. Sources of resistance to fumonisin accumulation in grain and Fusarium ear and kernel rot of corn. Phytopathology. 2004;**94**:251-260

[12] He X, Singh PK, Duveiller E, Schlang N, Dreisigacker S, Singh RP. Identification and characterization of international Fusarium head blight screening nurseries of wheat at CIMMYT, Mexico. European Journal of Plant Pathology. 2013;**136**:123-134

[13] Mesterhazy A, Lemmens M, Reid LM. Breeding for resistance to ear rots caused by *Fusarium* spp. in maize—A review. Plant Breeding. 2012;**131**:1-19

[14] Hart LP, Gendloff E, Rossman EC. Effect of corn genotypes on ear rot infection by *Gibberella zeae*. Plant Disease. 1984;**68**:296-298

[15] Pérez-Brito D, Jeffers D, González-de-León D, Khairallah M, Cortés-Cruz M, Velázquez-Cardelas G, Azpíroz-Rivero S, Srinivasan G. QTL mapping of *Fusarium moniliforme* ear rot resistance in highland maize. México. Agrociencia. 2001;**35**:181-196

[16] Robertson-Hoyt LA, Jines MP, Balint-Kurti PJ, Kleinschmidt CE, White DG, Payne GA, Maragos CM, Molnár TL, Holland JB. QTL mapping for Fusarium ear rot and fumonisin contamination resistance in two maize populations. Crop Science. 2006;**46**:1734-1743

[17] Reid LM, Zhu CX, Parker CA, Yan CW. Increased resistance to *Ustilago zeae* and *Fusarium verticillioides* in maize inbred lines bred for *Fusarium graminearum* resistance. Euphytica. 2009;**165**:567-578

[18] Shelby R, White DG, Burke EM. Differential fumonisin production in maize hybrids. Plant Disease. 1994;**78**:582-584

[19] de la Campa R, Hooker DC, Miller JD, Schaafsma AW, Hammond BG. Modeling effects of environment, insect damage, and Bt genotypes on fumonisin accumulation in maize in Argentina and the Philippines. Mycopathologia 2005;**159**:539-552

[20] Cao A, Santiago R, Ramos AJ, Souto XC, Aquin O, Malvar RA, Butron A. Critical environmental and genotypic factors for *Fusarium verticillioides* infection, fungal growth and fumonisin contamination in maize grown in northwestern Spain. International Journal of Food Microbiology. 2014;**177**:63-71

[21] Clements MJ, White DG. Identifying sources of resistance to aflatoxin and fumonisin contamination in corn grain. Journal of Toxicology-Toxin Reviews. 2004;**23**:381-396

[22] Eller M, Robertson-Hoyt LA, Payne GA, Holland JB. Grain yield and Fusarium ear rot of maize hybrids developed from lines with varying levels of resistance. Maydica. 2008;**53**:231-237

[23] Steiner B, Buerstmayr M, Michel S, Schweiger W, Lemmens M, Buerstmayr H. Breeding strategies and advances in line selection for Fusarium head blight resistance in wheat. Tropical Plant Pathology. 2017;**42**:165-174

[24] Hung H-Y, Holland JB. Diallel analysis of resistance to Fusarium ear rot and fumonisin contamination in maize. Crop Science. 2012;**52**:2173-2181

[25] Henry WB, Williams WP, Windham GL, Hawkins LK. Evaluation of maize inbred lines for resistance to Aspergillus and Fusarium ear rot and mycotoxin accumulation. Agronomy Journal. 2009;**101**:1219-1226

[26] Naidoo G, Forbes AM, Paul C, White DG, Rocheford TR. Resistance to *Aspergillus* ear rot and aflatoxin accumulation in maize F1 hybrids. Crop Science. 2002;**42**:360-364

[27] Reid LM, Bolton AT, Hamilton RI, Woldemariam T, Mather DE. Effect of silk age on resistance of maize to *Fusarium graminearum*. Canadian Journal of Plant Pathology. 1992;**14**:293-298

[28] Malla S, Ibrahim AMH, Glover KD. Diallel analysis of Fusarium head blight resistance in wheat. Journal of Crop Improvement. 2009;**23**:213-234

[29] Malla S, Ibrahim AMH, Glover KD, Berzonsky WA. Combining ability for fusarium head blight resistance in wheat (*Triticum aestivum* L.) Communications in Biometry and Crop Science. 2010;**5**(2):116-126

[30] Mardi M, Buerstmayr H, Ghareyazie B, Lemmens M, Moshrefzadeh N, Ruckenbauer P. Combining ability analysis of resistance to head blight caused by Fusarium graminearum in spring wheat. Euphytica. 2004;**139**(1):45-50

[31] Eller MS, Payne GA, Holland JB. Selection for reduced Fusarium ear rot and fumonisin content in advanced backcross maize lines and their topcross hybrids. Crop Science. 2010;**50**:2249-2260

[32] Ding J-Q, Wang X, Chander S, Yan J, Li J. QTL mapping of resistance to Fusarium ear rot using a RIL population in maize. Molecular Breeding. 2008;**22**:395-403

[33] Li Z, Ding J, Wang R, Chen J, Sun X, Chen W, Song W, Dong H, Dai X, Xia Z, Wu J. A new QTL for resistance to Fusarium ear rot in maize. Journal of Applied Genetics. 2011;**52**:403-406

[34] Chen J, Ding J, Li H, Li Z, Sun X, Li J, Wang R, Dai X, Dong H, Song W, Chen W, Xia Z, Wu J. Detection and verification of quantitative trait loci for resistance to Fusarium ear rot in maize. Molecular Breeding. 2012;**30**:1649-1656

[35] Zila CT, Samayoa LF, Santiago R, Butron A, Holland JB. A genome-wide association study reveals genes associated with Fusarium ear rot resistance in a maize core diversity panel. Genes, Genomes, and Genetics. 2013;**3**:2095-2104

[36] Maschietto V, Colombi C, Pirona R, Pea G, Strozzi F, Marocco A, Rossini L, Lanubile A. QTL mapping and candidate genes for resistance to Fusarium ear rot and fumonisin contamination in maize. BMC Plant Biology. 2017;**17**:20

[37] Xiang K, Zhang ZM, Reid LM, Zhu XY, Yuan GS, Pan GT. A meta-analysis of QTL associated with ear rot resistance in maize. Maydica. 2010;**55**:281-290

[38] Robertson-Hoyt LA, Betran J, Payne GA, White DG, Isakeit T, Maragos CM, Molnar TL, Holland JB. Relationships among resistances to Fusarium and Aspergillus ear rots and contamination by fumonisin and aflatoxin in maize; 2007;**97**:311-317

[39] Del Blanco IA, Frohberg RC, Stack RW, Berzonsky WA, Kianian SF. Detection of QTL linked to Fusarium head blight resistance in Sumai 3-derived North Dakota bread wheat lines. Theoretical and Applied Genetics. 2003;**106**:1027-1031

[40] Zhou WC, Kolb FL, Bai GH, Domier LL, Boze LK, Smith NJ. Validation of a major QTL for scab resistance with SSRmarkers and use of marker-assisted selection in wheat. Plant Breeding. 2003;**122**:40-46

[41] Miedaner T, Wilde F, Steiner B, Buerstmayr H, Korzun V, Ebmeyer E. Stacking quantitative trait loci (QTL) for Fusarium head blight resistance from non-adapted sources in an European elite spring wheat background and assessing their effects on deoxynivalenol (DON) content and disease severity. Theoretical and Applied Genetics. 2006;**112**:562-569

[42] Anderson JA. Marker-assisted selection for Fusarium head blight resistance in wheat. International Journal of Food Microbiology. 2007;**119**:51-53

[43] Wilde F, Korzun V, Ebmeyer E, Geiger HH, Miedaner T. Comparison of phenotypic and marker-based selection for Fusarium head blight resistance and DON content in spring wheat. Molecular Breeding. 2007;**19**:357-370

[44] von der Ohe C, Ebmeyer E, Korzun V, Miedaner T. Agronomic and quality performance of winter wheat backcross populations carrying non-adapted Fusarium head blight resistance QTL. Crop Science 2010;**50**:2283-2290

[45] Salameh A, Buerstmayr M, Steiner B, Neumayer A, Lemmens M, Buerstmayr H. Effects of introgression of two QTL for Fusarium head blight resistance from Asian spring wheat by marker assisted backcrossing into European winter wheat on Fusarium head blight resistance, yield and quality traits. Molecular Breeding. 2011;**28**:485-494

[46] Agostinelli AM, Clark AJ, Brown-Guedira G, Van Sanford DA. Optimizing phenotypic and genotypic selection for Fusarium head blight resistance in wheat. Euphytica. 2012;**186**:115-126

[47] Balut AL, Clark AJ, Brown-Guedira G, Souza E, Van Sanford DA. Validation of Fhb1 and QFhsnau-2DL in several soft red winter wheat populations. Crop Science 2013;**53**:934-945

[48] Duvick J. Prospects for reducing fumonisin contamination of maize through genetic modification. Environmental Health Perspective. 2001;**109**:337-342

[49] Yoneyama K, Anzai H. Gene technological study on disease-control by the inactivation of pathogenic toxins in transgenic plants. Journal of Pesticide Science. 1991;**16**:291-299

[50] Lu G, Scelonge C, Wang L, Norian L, Mancl M, Parson M, Cole G, Yalpani N, Bao A, Hu X, Heller J, Kulisek E, Schmidt H, Tagliani L, Duvick J, Bidney DL. Expression of oxalate oxidase in sunflower to combat *Sclerotinia* disease. Proceedings of the 1998 International Sclerotinia workshop; Fargo; 1998. p. 43

[51] Zhang L, Xu J, Birch R. Engineered detoxification confers resistance against a pathogenic bacterium. Nature Biotechnology. 1999;**17**:1021-1024

[52] Brown RL, Chen ZY, Cleveland TE, Russin JS. Advances in the development of host resistance in corn to aflatoxin contamination by *Aspergillus flavus*. Phytopathology. 1999;**89**:113-117

[53] Okubara PA, Blechl AE, Mccormick SP, Alexander NA, Dill-Macky R, Hohn TM. Engineering deoxynivalenol metabolism in wheat through the expression of a fungal trichothecene acetyltransferase gene. Theoretical and Applied Genetics. 2002;**106**:74-83

[54] Munkvold GP, Hellmich RL, Rice LG. Comparison of fumonisin concentrations in kernels of transgenic Bt maize hybrids and nontransgenic hybrids. Plant Disease. 1999;**83**:130-138

[55] Abbas HK, Zablotowicz RM, Weaver MA, Shier WT, Bruns HA, Bellaloui N, Accinelli C, Abel CA. Implications of Bt traits on mycotoxin contamination in maize: Overview and recent experimental results in southern United States. Journal of Agricultural and Food Chemistry. 2013;**61**:11759-11770

[56] Munkvold GP. Epidemiology of *Fusarium* diseases and their mycotoxins in maize ears. European Journal of Plant Pathology. 2003a;**109**:705-713

[57] Yadav A, Singh B, Sharma DK, Ahuja S. Effects of gamma irradiation on germination and physiological parameters of maize (*Zea mays*) genotypes. Indian Journal of Agricultural Sciences. 2015;**85**:1148-1152

[58] Borzouei A, Kafi M, Khazaei H, Naseriyan B, Majdabadi A. Effects of gamma radiation germination and physiological aspects of wheat (*Triticum aestivum* L.) seedlings. Pakistan Journal of Botany. 2010;**42**:281-290

[59] Khawar A, Bhatti IA, Khan QM, Bhatti HN, Sheikh MA. A germination test: An easy approach to know the irradiation history of seeds. Pakistan Journal of Agricultural Science. 2010;**47**:279-285

[60] Noreen Z, Ashraf M. Changes in antioxidant enzymes and some key metabolites in some genetically diverse cultivars of radish (*Raphanus sativus* L.). Environmental Experimental Botany. 2009;**67**:395-402

[61] Mashev N, Vassilev G, Ivanov K. A study of N-allyl N-2 pyridyl thiourea and gamma radiation treatment on growth and quality of peas and wheat. Bulgarian Journal of Plant Physiology. 1995;**21**:56-63

[62] Jain SM. Mutagenesis in crop improvement under the climate change. Romanian Biotechnological Letters. 2010;**15**:88-106

[63] Tomlekova NB. Induced mutagenesis for crop improvement in Bulgaria. Plant Mutation Reports. 2010;**2**:4-27

[64] Munkvold GP, Desjardins AE. Fumonisins in maize: Can we reduce their occurrence? The American Phytopathology Society. 1997;**81**:556-565

[65] Rheeder JP, Marasas WFO, Van Wyk PS, Van Schalkwyk DJ. Reaction of south African maize cultivars to ear inoculation with *Fusarium moniliforme, F. graminearum* and *Diplodia maydis*. Phytophylactica 1990;**22**:213-218

[66] Janse van Rensburg B, Mclaren NW, Flett BC, Schoeman A. Fumonisin producing *Fusarium* spp. and fumonisin contamination in commercial south African maize. European Journal of Plant Pathology. 2015;**141**:491-504

[67] Schjøth JE, Tronsmo AM, Sundheim L. Resistance to *Fusarium verticillioides* in 20 Zambian Maize Hybrids. Journal of Phytopathology. 2008;**156**:470-479

[68] Afolabi CG, Ojiambo PS, Ekpo EJA, Menkir A, Bandyopadhyay R. Evaluation of maize inbred lines for resistance to Fusarium ear rot and fumonisin accumulation in grain in tropical Africa. Plant Disease. 2007;**91**:279-286

[69] Small IM, Flett BC, Marasas WFO, McLeod A, Stander MA, Viljoen A. Resistance in maize inbred lines to *Fusarium verticillioides* and fumonisin accumulation in South Africa. Plant Disease. 2012;**96**:881-888

[70] Balconi C, Berardo N, Locatelli S, Lanzanova C, Torri A, Redaelli R. Evaluation of ear rot (Fusarium verticillioides) resistance and fumonisin accumulation in Italian maize inbred lines. Phytopathologica Mediterranea. 2014;**53**:14-26

[71] Rose LJ, Mouton M, Beukes I, Flett BC, van der Vyver C, Viljoen A. Multi-environment evaluation of maize inbred lines for resistance to Fusarium ear rot and fumonisins. Plant Disease. 2016;**100**:2134-2144

[72] Rose LJ, Okoth S, Beukes I, Mouton M, Flett BC, Makumbi D, Viljoen A. Determining resistance to *Fusarium verticillioides* and fumonisin accumulation in maize inbred lines resistant to *Aspergillus flavus* and aflatoxins. Euphytica. 2017;**213**:93. DOI: 10.1007/s10681-017-1883-7

[73] Okoth S, Rose LJ, Ouko A, Beukes I, Sila H, Mouton M, Flett BC, Makumbi D, Viljoen A. Field evaluation of resistance to aflatoxin accumulation in maize inbred lines in Kenya and South Africa. Journal of Crop Improvement. 2017a;**31**:862-878. DOI: 10.1080/15427528.2017.1391915

[74] Okoth S, Rose LJ, Ouko A, Nakisani NEI, Sila H, Viljoen A. Assessing genotype by environment interactions in Aspergillus ear rot and preharvest aflatoxin accumulation in maize inbred lines. Agronomy. 2017b;**7**:86

[75] Munkvold GP. Cultural and genetic approaches to managing mycotoxins in maize. Annual Review of Phytopathology. 2003b;**41**:99-116

[76] Blandino M, Reyneri A, Vanara F. Effect of plant density on toxigenic fungal infection and mycotoxin contamination of maize kernels. Field Crops Research. 2008a;**106**:234-241

[77] Abbas HK, Mascagni Jr HJ, Bruns HA, Shier WT, Damann KE. Effect of planting density, irrigation regimes, and maize hybrids with varying ear size on yield and aflatoxin and fumonisin contamination levels. American Journal of Plant Sciences. 2012;**3**:1341-1354

[78] Mukanga M, Derera J, Tongoona P. Gene action and reciprocal effects for ear rot resistance in crosses derived from five tropical maize populations. Euphytica. 2011;**174**:293-301

[79] Chulze SN, Ramirez ML, Farnochi MC, Pascale M, Visconti A, March G. *Fusarium* and fumonisin occurrence in Argentina corn at different ear maturity stages. Journal of Agricultural and Food Chemistry. 1996;**44**:2797-2801

[80] Bush BJ, Carson ML, Cubeta MA, Hagler WM, Payne GA. Infection and fumonisin production by *Fusarium verticillioides* in developing maize kernels. Phytopathology. 2004;**94**:88-93

[81] Flett BC. The potential of crop rotation in the control of maize ear and stalk rots caused by *Stenocarpella maydis*. Phytophylactica. 1993;**25**:184

[82] Marocco A, Gavazzi C, Pietri A, Tabaglio V. On fumonisin incidence in monoculture maize under no-till, conventional tillage and two nitrogen fertilisation levels. Journal of the Science of Food and Agriculture. 2008;**88**:1217-1221

[83] Gilbert J, Tekauz A. Strategies for management of Fusarium head blight (FHB) in cereals prairie soils. Crops J. 2011;**4**:97-104

[84] Magan N, Olsen M. Mycotoxins in Food: Detection and Control. CRC Press. Woodhead Publishing Limited; 2004. DOI: 10.1201/9781439823361

[85] Blandino M, Pilati A, Reyneri A, Scudellari D. Effect of maize crop residue density on Fusarium head blight and on deoxynivalenol contamination of common wheat grains. Cereal Research Communications. 2010;**38**(4):550-559. DOI: 101556/CRC382010412

[86] Flett BC. Crop rotation and tillage effects on yield and the incidence of root and stalk rot in sorghum (*Sorghum bicolor*). South African Journal of Plant and Soil. 1996;**13**:136-138

[87] Flett BC, Wehner FC. Incidence of Stenocarpella and Fusarium cob rots in monoculture maize under different tillage systems. Journal of Phytopathology. 1991;**133**:327-333

[88] Flett BC, Mclaren NW, Wehner FC. Incidence of ear rot pathogens under alternating corn tillage practices. Plant Disease. 1998;**82**:781-784

[89] McMullen M. An integrated approach to cereal disease management. In: Proceedings of the Manitoba-North Dakota Zero Tillage Farmer's Association 24th Annual Meeting; Minot, North Dakota; 2002. 1-5 pp

[90] Blandino M, Reyneri A, Vanara F. Influence of nitrogen fertilization on mycotoxin contamination of maize kernels. Crop Protection. 2008b;**27**:222-230

[91] Parsons MW, Munkvold GP. Associations of planting date, drought stress, and insects with Fusarium ear rot and fumonisin B1 contamination in California maize. Food Additives Contaminants: Part A. 2010;**27**:591-607

[92] Arino A, Juan T, Estopanan G, Gonzalez-Cabo JF. Natural occurrence of *Fusarium* species, fumonisin production by toxigenic strains, and concentrations of fumonisins B-1 and B-2 in conventional and organic maize grown in Spain. Journal of Food Protection. 2007;**70**:151-156

[93] de Galarreta JIR, Butrón A, Ortiz-Barredo A, Malvar RA, Ordás A, Landa A, Revilla P. Mycotoxins in maize grains grown in organic and conventional agriculture. Food Control 2015;**52**:98-102

[94] Miller JD. Factors that affect the occurrence of fumonisin. Environmental Health Perspectives. 2001;**109**:321-241

[95] Abbas HK, Cartwright RD, Xie W, Shier WT. Aflatoxin and fumonisin contamination of corn (maize, *Zea mays*) hybrids in Arkansas. Crop Protection. 2006;**25**:1-9

[96] Edwards SG, Pirgozliev SR, Hare MC, Jenkinson P. Quantification of trichothecene-producing *Fusarium* species in harvested grain by competitive PCR to determine the efficacy of fungicides against Fusarium head blight of winter wheat. Applied and Environmental Microbiology. 2001;**67**:1575-1580

[97] Nel A, Krause M, Khelawanlall N. A guide for the control of plant diseases. National Department of Agriculture, Pretoria, South Africa. 2003;131 pp

[98] Formenti Magan N, Pietri A, Battilani P. In vitro impact on growth, fumonisins and aflatoxins production by Fusarium verticillioides and Aspergillus flavus using anti-fungal compounds and a biological control agent. Phytopathologia Mediterranea. 2012;**51**:247-256

[99] Janse van Rensburg B. Modelling the incidence of *Fusarium* and *Aspergillus* toxin producing species in maize and sorghum in South Africa [PhD thesis]. Bloemfontein, South Africa: University of the Free State; 2012

[100] Forrer HR, Hecker A, Musa T, Schwab F, Bucheli TD, Wettstein FE, Vogelgsang S. Fusarium head blight control and prevention of mycotoxin contamination in wheat with botanicals and tannic acid. Toxins. 2014;**6**:830-849. DOI: 10.3390/toxins6030830

[101] Kumar A, Shukla R, Singh P, Prasad CS, Dubey NK. Assessment of *Thymus vulgaris* L. essential oil as a safe botanical preservative against post-harvest fungal infestation of food commodities. Innovative Food Science and Emerging Technologies. 2008;**9**:575-580. DOI: 10.1016/j.ifset.2007.12.005

[102] Sampietro DA, Fauguel CM, Vattuone MA, Presello DA, Catalan CAN. Phenylpropanoids from maize pericarp: Resistance factors to kernel infection and fumonisin accumulation by *Fusarium verticillioides*. European Journal of Plant Pathology. 2013;**135**:105-113

[103] Desjardins AE, Plattner RD, Lu M, Claflin LE. Distribution of fumonisins in maize ears infected with strains of *Fusarium moniliforme* that differ in fumonisin production. Plant Disease. 1998;**82**:953-958

[104] Luongo L, Galli M, Corazza L, Meekes E, de Haas L, Van Der Plas C, Köhl J. Potential of fungal antagonists for biocontrol of *Fusarium* spp. in wheat and maize through competition in crop debris. Biocontrol Science and Technology 2005;**15**:229-242

[105] Dorner JW, Cole RJ, Blackenship PD. Effect of inoculum rate of biological control agents on preharvest aflatoxin contamination of peanuts. Biological Control. 1998;**12**:171-176

[106] Bacon CW, Yates IE, Hinton DM, Meredith F. Biological control of *Fusarium moniliforme* in maize. Environmental Health Perspectives. 2001;**109**:325-332

[107] Benítez T, Rincón MA, Limón MC, Codón CA. Biocontrol mechanisms of *Trichoderma* strains. International microbiology. 2004;**7**:249-260

[108] Madden LV, Hughes G, van den Bosch F. The Study of Plant Disease Epidemics. The American Phytopathological Society; 2007:33-61. DOI.org/10.1094/9780890545058.003

[109] Van Maanen A, Xu XM. Modelling plant disease epidemics. European Journal of Plant Pathology. 2003;**109**:669-682

[110] Van der Plank JE. Analysis of epidemics. In: Horsfall JG, Cowling EB, editors. Plant Pathology: An Advanced Treatise. New York, USA: Academic Press; 1960. pp. 229-289

[111] Van der Plank JE. Plant Diseases: Epidemics and Control. New York, USA: Academic Press; 1963

[112] Schaafsma AW, Hooker DC. Climatic models to predict occurrence of *Fusarium* toxins in wheat and maize. International Journal of Food Microbiology. 2007;**119**:116-125

[113] De Wolf ED, Madden LV, Lipps PE. Risk assessment models for wheat Fusarium head blight epidemics based on within-season weather data. Phytopathology. 2003;**93**:248-435

[114] Musa T, Hecker A, Vogelsang S, Forrer HR. Forecasting of Fusarium head blight and deoxynivalenol content in winter wheat with FusaProg. Bulletin OEPP/EPPO. 2007;**37**:283-289

[115] Parsons MW, Munkvold GP. Effects of planting date and environmental factors on Fusarium ear rot symptoms and fumonisin B1 accumulation in maize grown in six north American locations. Plant Pathology; 2012;**61**:1130-1142. DOI: 10.1111/j.1365-3059.2011.02590.x

[116] Logrieco A, Mule G, Moretti A, Bottalico A. Toxigenic *Fusarium* species and mycotoxins associated with maize ear rot in Europe. European Journal of Plant Pathology. 2002;**108**:597-609

[117] Stewart DW, Reid LM, Nicol RW, Schaafsma AW. A mathematical simulation of growth of *Fusarium* in maize ears after artificial inoculation. Phytopathology. 2002;**92**:534-541

[118] Maiorano A, Reyneri A, Sacco D, Magni D, Ramponi C. A dynamic risk assessment model (FUMAgrain) of fumonisin synthesis by *Fusarium verticillioides* in maize grain in Italy. Crop Protection. 2009;**28**:243-256

Chapter 4

Biological Control of Mycotoxigenic Fungi and Their Toxins: An Update for the Pre-Harvest Approach

Mohamed F. Abdallah, Maarten Ameye,
Sarah De Saeger, Kris Audenaert and
Geert Haesaert

Additional information is available at the end of the chapter

http://dx.doi.org/10.5772/intechopen.76342

Abstract

Over recent decades, laboratory and field trial experiments have generated a considerable amount of data regarding the promising use of beneficial microorganisms to control plant diseases. Special attention has been paid to diseases caused by mycotoxigenic fungi owing to their direct destructive effect on crop yield and the potential production of mycotoxins, which poses a danger to animal and human health. New legislative initiatives to restrict the use of the existing commercial chemical pesticides have been an incentive for developing and registering new bio-pesticides. In this book chapter, we discuss up to-date pre-harvest biological control agents against mycotoxigenic fungi and their respective toxins. We will focus on the different modes of action of the most frequently studied biological control agents. Furthermore, a comprehensive overview on their ability to suppress mycotoxin biosynthesis will be discussed.

Keywords: biological control, mycotoxigenic fungi, mycotoxins, pre-harvest

1. State of the art

Cereals are a major source of calories consumed by people worldwide on a daily basis. With increasing global population, food production needs to increase by 50 to 70% in the next 30 years to avoid global food insecurity [1]. The danger of food insecurity is particularly serious for the developing countries especially sub-Saharan Africa where more people are suffering from hunger and this situation is expected to deteriorate in the future [2]. The challenge of safely and securely feeding these people, has to be faced in a world with a shrinking arable land, with less and more expensive fossil fuels, increasingly limited supplies of water, social unrest, economic uncertainty and within a scenario of a rapidly changing climate. Moreover the impact of plant diseases cannot be overestimated. The impact of fungal diseases and new variants of existing pathogens on agriculturally important crops is considered to be one of the main threats to worldwide food availability and safety. It was figured that diseases on our most important agricultural crops resulted in damages that were enough to feed 8.5% of the world's population [3]. The mission of providing food to the growing world population can therefore not be accomplished without a good control of these plant diseases. An important group of plant pathogens are toxigenic plant pathogens which produce mycotoxins, secondary metabolites of unrelated chemical structures and biological properties with a very broad toxic effects to humans and livestock, so in addition to posing a threat for food security, these pathogens also pose a threat to food safety [4–6].

Management of plant diseases can be done by adopting several strategies such as the cultivation of resistant cultivars, the use of sound crop rotation schemes and the use of chemical control. The harmful impact of plant protection products on the environment and human and animal health have prompted the European Union (EU Directive 2009/128/EC) to encourage research on alternative and ecofriendly solutions such as integrated pest management and the use of biological control agents (BCAs). Biological control, henceforth called biocontrol, in plant pathology, aims at utilizing microorganisms to prevent the colonization and/or suppress the spread of harmful plant pathogens [7]. BCAs in this chapter are defined as beneficial microorganisms that are able to antagonize plant pathogens and protect the plant [8–11]. Although the definition includes both pre-harvest and post-harvest strategies, this chapter will focus on pre-harvest biocontrol measures [12, 13].

The most studied mycotoxin producing plant pathogenic genera are *Fusarium, Alternaria, Claviceps, Stachybotrys* and *Aspergillus* spp. [4, 14–16]. These genera infect a wide array of commodities including cereals, nuts, beans, sugarcane, and sugar beet in the field (e.g. *Fusarium, Alternaria* and *Claviceps* spp.*)* and/or during storage (e.g. *Aspergillus* spp.). **Figure 1** illustrates, in term of biological control, the most studied mycotoxigenic fungi in pre-harvest in different crops. *Fusarium graminearum* is a predominant pathogen in wheat and maize, *Fusarium verticillioides* contaminates maize while *Aspergillus flavus* infects groundnuts and maize. Other mycotoxigenic plant pathogens such *Alternaria alternata, Claviceps purpurea,* and other members of the genera *Fusarium* (e.g. *F. avenaceum, F. acuminatum,* and *F. proliferatum*) and *Aspergillus* (e.g. *A. carbonarius, A. niger, and A. parasiticus*) received less attention in research to date.

Mycotoxins are ubiquitous in agricultural crops and their production occurs under certain environmental conditions during and/or after plant colonization [4, 17]. Exposure to mycotoxins either in a short and/or long term can lead to diverse toxic effects on a wide range of organisms [5, 6, 14, 17, 18]. Often, these fungal toxins are not only harmful for vertebrates and invertebrates (mycotoxins) but also for plants (phytotoxins). Economically, these natural contaminants hamper the international trade and significantly affect the world economy

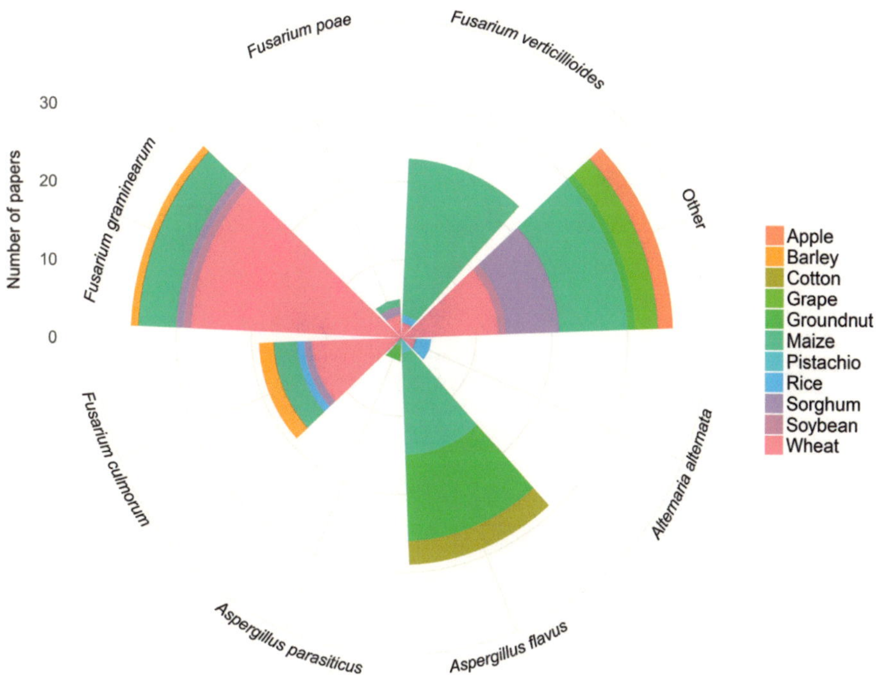

Figure 1. Overview of the number of papers published between 1989 and 2017 which use biological control strategies against, mycotoxigenic plant pathogenic fungi in different crops.

due to borders rejection when mycotoxin concentrations exceed the maximum permissible levels. Although the production of mycotoxins by these toxigenic plant pathogens is of economic importance, many research groups do not take them into account when studying biological control strategies. These studies are then limited to the fungicidal or fungistatic effects of the BCAs while the effect of the BCAs on mycotoxin production is often overlooked. **Figure 2A** subscribes this issue and shows the number of papers on mycotoxigenic fungi with and without considering mycotoxins under *in vitro*, greenhouse and field conditions over the last 30 years. The figures presented in **Figure 2A** are even an underestimation, as they comprise research on *A. flavus* (**Figure 2B**). Many of these papers deal with "Aflasafe" and all include aflatoxin measurements. Omitting these *A. flavus* data provides a more correct view on the lack of studies investigating the effects of BCAs on mycotoxin production (**Figure 2C**).

In view of the importance of mycotoxins for animal and human health, this review will focus on the effect of BCAs on the mycotoxin production by toxigenic plant pathogenic fungi. In a first part, we will provide an overview on the diverse modes of action BCAs can have. Secondly, a more in depth insight into the effect of BCAs on production of the major mycotoxins is provided. Finally, we end by providing some perspectives for future research and hurdles that might have to be taken.

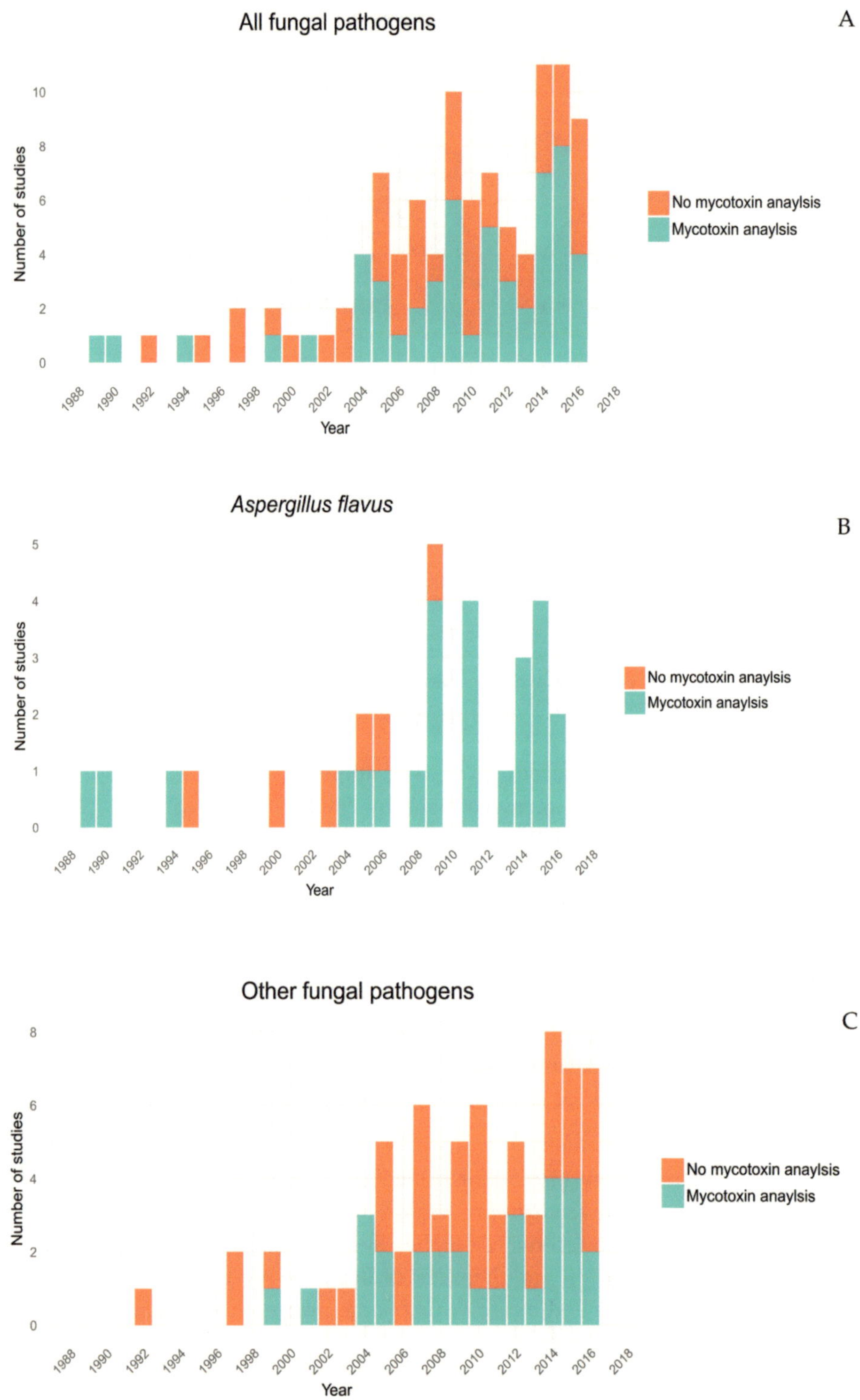

Figure 2. Number of published papers between the period of 1988–2017 addressing biocontrol of mycotoxigenic fungi with and without considering the effect on mycotoxins.

2. Modes of action of BACs

The main modes of action of BCAs are **antibiosis, competition, mycoparasitism**, and **stimulation or enhancement of plant defense** [7]. BCAs usually relay on more than one mode of action to antagonize the pathogen i.e. presence of one dominant mode of action does not exclude the others. **Table 1** summarizes the reported modes of action used against mycotoxigenic fungi in each crop.

(i) **Antibiosis** encompasses the production of secondary metabolites such as antibiotics [19–21], lytic enzymes [22] and other proteins [23] that are able to suppress the growth, weaken the virulence or kill the pathogenic fungi.

(ii) **Competition** occurs when two or more fungi compete for the same essential nutrients required for their growth and development [24, 25]. Another type of competition is exclusion by occupying the same niche [26, 27].

(iii) **Mycoparasitism** or **hyperparasitism** is a direct parasitic attack of one fungus by another one which eventually causes death of the host pathogen [28–30].

(iv) **Colonization of the plant**, by beneficial micro-organisms can trigger local or systemic defense responses, thus enhancing resistance against plant pathogens [31, 32].

2.1. Antibiosis

Production of a wide range of antibiotics, enzymes and other antifungal compounds which contribute to adverse impacts on plant pathogen are characteristic features of different fungal BCAs such as *Trichoderma* spp. and *Clonostachys* spp. [8, 11, 24, 33]; bacterial BCAs such as *Bacillus* spp., *Pseudomonas* spp., *Streptomyces* spp. and *Lactobacillus* spp. [19, 20, 34, 35]; and yeast BCAs such as *Cryptococcus* spp., *Kluyveromyces* spp. and *Saccharomyces* spp. [10, 36]. All these BCAs have an arsenal of metabolites targeting different structures of the pathogen which thereafter curtails the growth or kills the pathogen.

A. Enzymes hydrolyzing fungal cell wall

The fungal cell wall is a complex structure containing mainly glucan polymers and chitin. For several BCAs, molecules which interfere with this cell wall have been described. Peptaibols, linear oligopeptides produced by *Trichoderma* spp., inhibit beta-glucan synthase which prevents the pathogen from reconstructing its cell wall [37]. Culture filtrates of a *T. harzianum* isolate changed the colony color of *A. flavus* and had a clear effect on the growth. A microscope study showed alterations in the morphology of *A. flavus* represented by abnormal vesicle formation and various aberrant conidial heads reflecting cell wall deformity [38]. Production of some extracellular enzymes (amylolytic, cellulolytic, pectinolytic, lipolytic and proteolytic) were also demonstrated, however the inhibition was directly associated with source of carbon (glucose or sucrose) or nitrogen (L-alanine or other) available in the medium [38].

B. Production of metabolites that affect fungal membrane

Production of antifungal metabolites interfering with membrane structures have been described in several BCAs. The most important class is the lipopeptides which interfere with the membrane and the sterols in the membrane [39]. These lipopeptides have been proven to be effective against several genera of toxigenic fungi such as *Aspergillus* and *Fusarium* spp.

The presence of two antibiotic lipopeptides, iturin and surfactin, revealed the potent antifungal activity [20] of two *Bacillus* spp. (P1 and P11) against *A. flavus* [40]. Similarly, *B. subtilis* BS119m was able to completely inhibit *A. flavus* growth which was associated to its ability to produce a high amount of surfactin [41]. Crane et al. monitored iturins produced by *B. amyloliquefaciens* in wheat under greenhouse and the field conditions and found an inverse relationship between iturins levels and *Fusarium* disease incidence [42]. Fengycin, another lipopeptide purified from *Bacillus subtilis* IB culture showed an inhibitory effect against *F. graminearum* [19].

C. Production of antifungal compounds having antibiotic effects not related to membrane and cell wall effects

Where antibiotics have been described as powerful allies in the battle against bacterial contaminants, several molecules have been described which are fungicidal. The polyketide compound 2,4-diacetylphloroglucinol (DAPG) produced by *P. fluorescens* has received a particular consideration due to the broad spectrum activity against various fungal pathogens [43–46]. The molecule was isolated from *Pseudomonas* spp. strain F113 present in the rhizosphere of sugar beets [46] and has later been isolated from the rhizosphere of different crops [47]. DAPG has been shown to have antifungal effects against *Fusarium* and *Alternaria* spp. [48].

Although antibiosis has been proven to be a major weapon against plant pathogenic, fungal resistance might arise. One example is known for *F. verticillioides* in which a Lactamase encoding gene (FVEG_08291) has been identified which enables the pathogen to resist benzoxazinoid phytoanticipins produced in plant but also possibly microbial xenobiotic lactam compounds [49]. This information therefore raises an important question about the ability of mycotoxigenic plant pathogens to cope with the antifungal compounds produced by BCAs. In case that reported fungal resistance may be present against BCAs, this may necessitate the continuous exploration of new antibiotics.

2.2. Competition for niche and nutrition

Competition for niche or competitive exclusion is a restriction of access to the habitat of a pathogen on the plant or seeds by another microorganism while competition for nutrients happens when two or more microorganisms compete for the same source of macro- and micro-nutrients required for growth and secondary metabolites production [7].

One of the most famous and promising examples on competition for ecological niche and nutrition is found in *A. flavus* control [26]. However, competition of other mycotoxigenic pathogens such as *F. pseudograminearum* through nutrient competition [50] and *F. culmorum* and *F. graminearum* [51] were also reported. It has been demonstrated that atoxigenic *A. flavus* strains are powerful BCAs to control the toxigenic strains of *A. flavus* in cottonseed [52–54], maize [27, 55–57] and various types of nuts [58–61]. Currently, different strains of atoxigenic *A. flavus* are being used depending on the endemic area and sometimes a mixture of strains is used in the field. This competitive exclusion theory has been recently confirmed in situ by co-inoculating corn kernels with GFP-labeled AF70 and wild-type AF36. The study showed that there is a population difference (up to 82% reduction) between the co-inoculated kernels with both fungi and the control one inoculated only with GFP-labeled AF70 after visualizing under UV. Furthermore, aflatoxins (AFs) analysis showed a 73% reduction compared to the control [62].

However, AFs are not the only toxic compounds produced by *A. flavus*. Cyclopiazonic acid (CPA) is another mycotoxin produced by certain strains of *A. flavus*, including the atoxigenic strains, affecting mainly the liver and muscles of livestock [63, 64]. As an example, the commercially registered BCAs AF36, while it is effective against toxigenic *A. flavus*, it has been confirmed for its CPA production in cottonseeds. Therefore, researchers screened and tested new strains lacking the production of both toxins for the same previously mentioned crops [65–67]. Testing atoxigenic strains of *A. flavus* against other AFs producing fungi such as *A. parasiticus* was less common because *A. parasiticus* is less virulent and not predominantly occurs in the soil as *A. flavus* [59].

Competition for nutrient and niche can also be seen in *Trichoderma* and *Clonostachys* spp. when they are applied before pathogen occurrence [11, 68]. *Trichoderma* spp., especially *T. harzianum*, produce siderophores, low-molecular-mass ferric-iron-specific chelators, when the available iron in the environment is low [23]. Siderophores chelate the oxidized ferric ions (Fe + 3) making it available as an iron source [24, 37, 69] and this enables *Trichoderma* spp. to compete for iron which is an essential element for the development of many plant pathogens [24, 68].

2.3. Mycoparasitism

Mycoparasitism is a direct parasitic relationship between one fungus and another fungal host [24]. The mycoparasitic interaction is mediated through certain gene involved in synthesis of some metabolites (mainly chitinases, glucanases, and proteases) allowing the parasitic fungi to degrade and invade the host cells [24, 29, 70]. A wide array of BCAs employ this strategy to compete against several mycotoxigenic pathogens especially against *Fusarium* spp. Among these, *Trichoderma* spp., are a widespread mycoparasitic BCA naturally present in the soil and the plant [11, 70, 71]. The fungi are mainly biotrophic, perform mycoparasitic interaction with living fungi, although the species also compete for niche and nutrients, enhance the plant systemic and localized resistance and secrete secondary antifungal metabolites [29, 68]. Upregulation of some chitinase-encoding genes occurred upon mycoparasitic contact of *Trichoderma* spp. with *Fusarium* [71, 72]. *T. viride* showed a potent antagonisms of *F. verticillioides* in an *in vitro* assay which was proven by the suppression of radial extension of the fungus by 46% after 6 days and by 90% after 14 days [73].

On rice, *T. harzianum* performed very well against *F. verticillioides* through mycoparasitism and showed a mutual antagonism by contact [74]. Some metabolites such as cell wall-degrading enzymes, chitinases and ß-1,3 glucanases were suggested by the author to be involved in the mechanism as the evidence of mycoparasitism in this study was supported by cryo scanning electron microscopic observations. The same experimental setup was previously done using the same BCA on rice but against *Alternaria alternata* and similar results and conclusions were reported [75]. Upon fungal cell wall degradation by chitinases produced by *Trichoderma* spp., another type of enzymes called exochitinases are secreted and the attack starts to kill the pathogen [24].

Trichoderma spp. have mostly been tested as a BCA against *F. graminearum* in wheat [38, 51, 76–78]. In a field trial, T-22 strain, reduced formation of perithecia of *F. graminearum* by 70% [77].

Clonostachys is another genus famous for mycoparasitism and demonstrates a promising BCA against a wide range of plant pathogens including *F. graminearum, F. verticillioides, F. poae*, and *F. culmorum*. However, compared to *Trichoderma, Clonostachys* spp. are poorly studied. Within *Clonostachys* spp., *C. rosea* is the most researched and has been associated with multiple modes of action such as antibiosis [33], induction of plant resistance, [79], and niche and nutrient competition [80]. The fungus *C. rosea* secretes a number of antibiotics such as peptaibols, gliotoxin, trichoth as well as cell wall degrading enzymes such as chitinases, glucanases. *C. Rosa* ACM941 was reported to produce chitin-hydrolysing enzymes capable of degrading cell wall of *F. culmorum* [81].

Recently, *Sphaerodes* spp. have been discovered as a potential biocontrol agent against *Fusarium* spp. relying on mycoparasitism tactics with promising results. Among these species *Sphaerodes mycoparasitica* was isolated in association with *Fusarium* spp. from wheat and asparagus fields [82] and has shown its ability to limit *Fusarium* infection in both 3-ADON and 15-ADON chemotypes and limit DON synthesis both in vivo and in planta [82, 83]. For bacterial BCAs, Palumbo et al. [84] reported the production of antifungal metabolites and chitinase by *P. fluorescens* (strains JP2034 and JP2175) which had negative effects on the growth of *A. flavus* and *F. verticillioides*.

2.4. Indirect through the plant

Enhancement of systemic plant resistance using plant growth-promoting rhizobacteria, which results an effective protection against a broad spectrum of pathogens, has been well described [85–87]. *P. fluorescens* is known to produce various plant growth regulators such as indole acetic acid, gibberellins and cytokinins which interfere with plant signaling [88]. In addition, it also produces antibiotics, volatile compounds, enzymes [21, 89]. The production of indole-3-acetic acid by *P. fluorescens* MPp4 is triggered by the presence of some pathogens such as *F. verticillioides* M1 which in turn contributes into its antagonistic activity [90]. *P. fluorescens* CHA0 prevented the carbon diversion and plant biomass reduction due to *F. graminearum* infection in barley [91]. The antagonistic activity of *P. fluorescens* MKB158 against *F. culmorum* was documented by Khan et al., however, the author mentioned that an indirect effect through enhancement of the plant systemic resistant is involved in the antagonistic activity [92]. *Lysobacter enzymogenes* strain C3 exerts also its biocontrol effect though induction of resistance in wheat against *F. graminearum* beside the production of lytic enzymes [93]. Effective reduction of the pathogen after heat treatment of C3 broth cultures to inactivate the bacterial cells and lytic enzymes was a confirmation for the presence of some fungal elicitors.

Besides rhizobacteria, the fungus *T. harzianum*, while, has also been shown to promote plant growth, increase nutrient availability and enhance the resistance against fungal diseases through colonization of plant roots [24, 37, 70]. Extensive research has been done to use *Trichoderma* spp., against *F. verticillioides* [94], *F. graminearum* [78] and *A. flavus* [95]. *T. harzianum* was reported to limit *F. verticillioides* in maize through the induction of systemic resistance by inducing ethylene and jasmonate signaling pathways [96]. Recently, novel species of *Trichoderma* (*T. stromaticum, T. amazonicum, T. evansii, T. martiale, T. taxi* and *T. theobromicola)* are classified as true endophytes as they have been reported to invade the plant tissue away from the root and induce transcriptomic changes in plants and protect the plants from diseases and abiotic stresses [97].

Another approach to enhance the plant resistance is through colonization. Extensive research is being done to discover endophytic microorganisms which colonize plant (tissue) without harming the plant [98] to reduce the plant diseases and mycotoxins in crops [99–103]. Endophytes can enhance plant growth and fitness, and offer protection against biotic and abiotic stresses by inducing plant defense responses. However, it should be noted that some of them are pathogenic to the plant in some phases of their lifecycle or under certain environmental conditions [98]. Some endophytes exert its role to enhance the host immune system against several fungal pathogens through the improvement of the nutrient uptake from the soil such as *Piriformospora indica,* a cultivable root fungal endophyte belonging to the order Sebacinales in Basidiomycota [104, 105]. The ability of *Piriformospora indica* to protect barley from root rot caused by *F. graminearum* was confirmed [103]. This was supported by a positive correlation between the relative amount of fungal DNA and disease symptoms and the absence of an inhibition on the growth of *F. graminearum* when co-inoculated with *Piriformospora indica* in an *in vitro* assay. Another endophyte such as *Epicoccum nigrum* has also proven its biocontrol activity against several plant pathogens [106], however it is ability to control diseases caused by mycotoxin producing fungi were scarcely studied [107, 108].

			Mode of action of BCAs				
	Pathogen	**Host**	**Mycoparasitism**	**Antibiosis**	**Competition for niche / nutrients**	**Indirect through the plant**	**References**
Alternaria	*alternata*	Wheat	✓	✓	✓		[48, 107]
		Rice	✓	✓	✓		[75, 109]
Aspergillus	*terreusHAP1*	Apple	✓	✓	✓		[110]
	carbonarius	Grape		✓	✓		[111, 112]
	flavus	Cottonseed			✓		[52–54]
		Pistachio nuts		✓	✓		[113, 114]
		Peanuts	✓	✓	✓		[58–61, 66, 115–119]
		Maize	✓	✓	✓	✓	[27, 55, 56, 65, 67, 84, 95, 118, 120–124]
	niger	Peanuts		✓			[125]
		Grape		✓	✓		[111]
	parasiticus	Peanuts			✓		[59, 60]
Fusarium		Maize			✓		[121]
	acuminatum	Maize				✓	[126]
		Sorghum				✓	[126]

Pathogen	Host	Mode of action of BCAs				References
		Mycoparasitism	Antibiosis	Competition for niche / nutrients	Indirect through the plant	
	Wheat				✓	[126]
avenaceum	Maize				✓	[126]
	Sorghum				✓	[126]
	Wheat	✓	✓		✓	[126, 127]
culmorum	Barley		✓		✓	[92, 102]
	Maize	✓	✓			[72, 127–129]
	Wheat	✓	✓	✓	✓	[48, 51, 130–132]
	Rice	✓	✓	✓		[133]
equiseti	Maize				✓	[126]
	Sorghum				✓	[126]
	Wheat				✓	[126]
graminearum	Barley				✓	[103]
	Maize	✓	✓		✓	[99, 128, 129, 134]
	Sorghum				✓	[126]
	Wheat	✓	✓	✓	✓	[35, 48, 51, 72, 76–78, 89, 93, 100, 101, 107, 108, 126, 127, 129–131, 135–144]
	Soybean	✓	✓	✓		[145]
langsethiae	Wheat	✓	✓			[127]
nivale	Maize				✓	[126]
	Sorghum				✓	[126]
	Wheat				✓	[126]
poae	Maize					[126]
	Sorghum				✓	[126]
	Wheat	✓	✓	✓	✓	[107, 126, 127]
proliferatum	Maize	✓	✓			[129, 146]
	Wheat	✓	✓			[129]
sambucinum	Maize				✓	[126]
	Sorghum				✓	[126]
	Wheat				✓	[126]
sporotrichioides	Maize				✓	[126]
	Sorghum				✓	[126]
	Wheat	✓	✓		✓	[126, 127]
verticillioides	Rice	✓		✓		[74]
	Maize	✓	✓	✓	✓	[73, 84, 90, 94–96, 146–158]
	Wheat	✓	✓			[127]
crookwellense	Maize				✓	[126]
	Sorghum				✓	[126]
	Wheat	✓	✓		✓	[78, 126]

Table 1. Different modes of action used by BCAs against mycotoxigenic fungi.

3. Biocontrol and mycotoxins

3.1. Trichothecenes toxins

Fusarium head blight (FHB) and *Fusarium* ear rot (FER) are two of the most serious diseases affecting wheat and maize respectively throughout the world [130, 131, 139]. Over the last few years, FHB was predominantly caused by three species of *Fusarium*: *F. graminearum*, *F. avenaceum* and *F. culmorum* [108, 159] while FER is mainly caused by *F. verticillioides*, *F. proliferatum*, *F. subglutinans*, and *F. graminearum* [154, 156]. However FHB mostly occurs as a complex of several species [14, 160]. Each disease has multi-destructive effects on the crop through reducing the yield and grain quality. Over 180 types of trichothecenes are produced by *Fusarium* spp. contaminating mainly agricultural staples such as maize, wheat, and barley [14, 15]. The most prominent members are deoxynivalenol (DON), nivalenol (NIV) and T-2 Toxin. The biochemical importance of DON for fungal growth and development is not fully clear yet; however, it may have an important role during fungal infection and colonization and act as a virulence factor [160]. In animals, DON interferes with the cellular protein synthesis and clinically causing animal feed refusal and vomiting while NIV may induce genotoxic effect and leucopenia on long term exposure [4, 5, 17]. T-2 toxin triggers apoptosis to immune cells [161]. Due to the complexity of the life cycle of *Fusarium* spp., researchers mostly tried two application strategies to biologically control the disease, treatment of the crop residue with the antagonist or treatment of wheat ears at anthesis [162]. Most of the performed experiments used bacterial BCAs rely on antibiosis mainly to control the diseases and DON level. Less research discussed the effect of BCAs on NIV [51] and T-2 toxin [107].

An isolate of *Trichoderma*, *T. gamsii* 6085, was selected as a potential antagonist against *F. culmorum* and *F. graminearum*. The strain exhibited the capacity to negatively affect DON production by both pathogens up to 92% [72]. A field experiment on winter wheat for two seasons was conducted to evaluate the efficacy of different BCAs against ear blight and associated DON presence. Two strains of *F. equiseti* were the best performing strains and decreased the mycotoxins level produced by *F. culmorum* and *F. graminearum* by 70 and 94%, respectively. However, low levels of NIV in the cereals treated with *F. equiseti* were detected [51]. Recently, *Piriformospora indica* has proven its promising ability to reduce the severity the disease caused by *F. graminearum* and mycotoxin DON contamination in wheat by 70–80% and increase the total grain weight of *F. graminearum*-inoculated samples by 54% [100]. Novel bacterial endophytes predicted to be *Paenibacillus polymyxa* and *Citrobacter* were able to detoxify DON *in vitro*, but the performance of some of these isolated strains under field condition or in green house has not been reported yet [99].

Three stains of the yeast *Cryptococcus* spp. (*Cryptococcus nodaensis* OH182.9, *Cryptococcus* spp. OH 71.4, and *Cryptococcus* spp. OH 181.1) were tested in several field experiments and they could control the disease by 50–60% on susceptible winter wheat. However DON content was the same as control [137]. Later, the same group cultivated another strain, *Cryptococcus flavescens* OH 182.9, and applied it at early anthesis but found no effects on DON level [142].

Besides fungal and yeast BCAs, bacteria have also been used to control DON produced by *F. graminearum* in wheat [35, 139, 144, 163] and in maize [99]. A complete reduction in DON content was achieved when *B. subtilis* RC 218 and *Brevibacillus* spp. RC 263 were applied at anthesis for two seasons [144] which was consistent with previous findings under greenhouse conditions by the same authors [163], although there was no constant reduction in the disease incidence. Opposite to that, Khan and Doohan tested three strains of *Pseudomonas* spp., two strains of *fluorescens* and one strain of *frederiksbergensis*, against *F. culmorum* and DON production in wheat and barley in a small scale field experiment. The results showed that DON was reduced in wheat and barley by 12 and 21%, respectively [164].

Other types of trichothecenes were not well researched as the previously mentioned toxins due to their low incidence in crops. Variable results for T-2 toxin after spraying the ears of susceptible and resistant wheat cultivars with *Trichoderma* spp. under greenhouse conditions were documented. The author used four fungi, *Epicoccum* spp., *Trichoderma* spp., *Penicillium* spp. and *Alternaria* spp. however the last one is known for production of *Alternaria* toxins [107].

3.2. Zearalenone

Although zearalenone (ZEN) is an important mycotoxin in many cereals, less attention has been paid to control this toxin. ZEN is a potent mycoestrogen which competitively binds to estrogen receptors causing reproductive disorders in farm animals and human [5]. Other forms of ZEN include α and β zearalenol, zearalanone and, α and β –zearalanol which are often detected at variable concentration usually lower than ZEN.

Trichoderma isolates have recently been reported to detoxify ZEN by transforming ZEN into reduced and sulfated forms [165]. This was in accordance with previous results by Gromadzka et al. who tested two isolates of *Trichoderma* and several isolates of *Clonostachys in vitro* against two isolates of *F. graminearum* and two isolates of *F. culmorum*. Despite the high rate of ZEN reduction (over 96%), the performance of these isolates under greenhouse or field experiments was not confirmed [128].

C. rosea converts ZEN into less toxic compounds through an enzymatic alkaline hydrolysis by lactonohydrolase *in vitro* [23, 166]. This has been proved after cloning the coding region of the responsible gene, *zhd 101*, and expressing in *Schizosaccharomyces pombe* [167] and *Escherichia coli*, but not with *Saccharomyces cerevisiae* which exhibited weak detoxification activity against ZEN [168]. Through this approach which involves the direct interaction between BCAs and pathogen toxin, resistance of BCAs to mycotoxin itself is an important feature to ensure the efficacy and durability. Also, it was proven that *C. rosea* is tolerant to ZEN exposure due to the presence of high numbers of ATP-binding cassette transporters [169].

3.3. Fumonisins

Fumonisin B1 (FB1), the main member of fumonisins, is produced by *F. verticillioides* and *F. proliferatum* which usually infect maize [14]. The mycotoxin suppresses ceramide synthase and causes neurological toxicities in horses, pulmonary edema in pigs, and may pose hepatotoxicity and esophageal cancer in human [18]. Therefore, several trials have been conducted to effectively control the mycotoxin in maize using different strategies. Most of the field studies were done using bacterial BCAs [147, 148, 150, 158] while other types of BCAs, and fungi, were restricted to *in vitro* testing [73, 154–156]. Maize rhizobacterial isolates belonging to *Pseudomonas* and *Bacillus* genera significantly reduced the mycotoxin production by 70 to 100% [157]. However, in another study, a mixture of *P. Solanacearum* and *B. subtilis* was not able to affect FB1 concentration [151]. Seed treatment with *B. amyloliquefaciens* Ba-S13 was sufficient to reduce fumonisins B1 concentration in maize field tests [148]. That has been confirmed in a 2-year field study with the same bacteria, *B. amyloliquefaciens*, after application of two different treatments: inoculating seeds during pre-sowing and maize ears at flowering [150].

P. fluorescens isolated from maize rhizosphere by Nayaka et al. had a clear reduction of FB1 content and the disease incidence after challenge with *F. verticillioides* during a 3-years study [147]. Seed treatment followed by spray treatment with a pure culture of *P. fluorescens* reduced the incidence of fumonisins by 88% [147]. Bacon et al. suggested the use of the endophytic bacterium, *B. subtilis* to control FB1 production as a convenient approach to prevent the vertical transmission of the fungi. Under greenhouse conditions, FB1 was reduced by 50% [154].

When *T. viride* was co-inoculated in corn kernels with *F. verticillioides*, a reduction of FB1 by 72–85% was obtained depending on the time of inoculation [73]. The fungus was also proposed as a postharvest agent to prevent the accumulation of the toxins during storage [73, 154]. It was proven that *C. rosea* can inhibit the synthesis of fumonisins by *F. verticillioides* but does not degrade it [170]. Constant reduction of FB1 by 60–70% depending on the temperature when a 50:50 mixture of the pathogen and *C. rosea* 016 applied at different ripening stage of maize cobs. These investigations were done as *F. verticillioides* may attack maize at ripening under suitable environmental conditions [156]. Previously, similar results at the same concentration (50:50/ pathogen: *C. rosea* 016) in milled maize agar were also reported [155]. It could be concluded that using bacterial BCAs rely on antibiosis was more effective to control FB1 *in vitro* and in field trials.

3.4. Aflatoxins

AFs are the most natural carcinogenic substance in the history targeting mainly liver and are classified as Group 1 according to the International Agency for Research on Cancer [4, 6, 16, 171]. *A. flavus* and *A. parasiticus* infect mostly groundnuts, maize, cottonseed, soybean and tree nuts in the field and/or during storage producing a wide range of secondary toxic metabolites including AFs [60, 172]. Researchers have mostly been focusing on *A. flavus* as the fungus is highly invasive and more widespread in nature compared to *A. parasiticus*. Regarding their ability to synthetize mycotoxins, toxigenic *A. flavus* strains produce aflatoxin B1 (AFB1) and B2 (AFB2) while *A. parasiticus* produces four types of AFs (AFB1, AFB2, AFG1 and AFG2). CPA is only produced by *A. flavus* including strains which lack the potential to produce AFs [173].

In general, reduction of AFs in different crops has mostly been performed with non-toxigenic *A. flavus* strains [27, 52, 54, 60, 65, 114, 120, 123]. Some of these strains (AF36 as an example) are commercially available in the market [53, 65]. Two theories are suggested on the mode of action for the reduction of AFs by non-toxigenic *A. flavus* BCAs; (i) reduction due to competitive exclusion on toxigenic wild *A. flavus* population and (ii) inhibition of biosynthetic pathways involved in aflatoxin production, however the exact mechanism is still obscure [62].

Doster et al. used *A. flavus* strain AF36 as a BCA to control AFs in pistachio orchards for four consecutive seasons (2008–2011) and he could diminish AFs level by 20–45% [114]. In groundnuts, more trials *in vitro* [61, 66] and in the field [58–60] have been done. Zhou et al. 2015 found a positive correlation between AFs reduction rate and inoculum dose while Hulikunte Mallikarjunaiah et al. 2017 measured total AFs in rhizospheric and geocarpospheric soil and groundnut seeds after he treated them with two strains isolated from India. A significant reduction of mycotoxin concentration below the maximum permissible levels for ground nuts was obtained [61]. Field trials in Argentina were designed to control AFs in groundnut. However, the author reported a high level of AFs reduction, and the results were inconsistent between the two seasons [58, 59].

High levels of AFs and CPA control in maize field were achieved after challenging two strains of *A. flavus* with atoxigenic strains K49 and NRRL 21882 [65]. Mauro et al. could obtain similar results *in vitro* after screening for local atoxigenic strains from Italy [67]. In Nigeria, a successful maize field trial exhibited the promising use of two locally isolated strains, La3279 and La3303, in controlling AFB1 and AFB2 up to 99.9% [120]. When these two strains mixed with other two strains to make a mixture applied to the soil before flowering, a similar conclusion was obtained [55] with the advantage of persistence of the biocontrol effect during storage.

Researchers have also tested different species of *Trichoderma* such as *T. viride*, *T. harzianum* and *T. asperellum* [38, 95, 115, 116]; bacteria [84, 121, 124]; yeast [36, 174]; and algae [118] as a potential alternative BCAs to control *Aspergillus* spp., although not all have looked into mycotoxins (**Figure 2B**). Production of two volatile compounds, dimethyl trisulfide and 2,4-bis(1,1-dimethylethyl)-phenol, by *Shewanella algae* strain YM8 showed a 100% inhibition on aflatoxin synthesis in maize and peanuts stored at different water activities [118]. Previously, *B. subtilis* RCB 90 *in vitro* was also reported to completely inhibit AFB1 [121]. The yeast, *Candida parapsilosis* IP1698 was also able to inhibit aflatoxin production (90–99%) at different pH and temperatures [174]. This was also in line with the same reduction percentage obtained but with *Bacillus* spp. P1 and *Bacillus* spp. P11 [40]. Aiyaz et al. tested in the field, four BCAs and all the formulations, by maize seeds treatment application, had a significant reduction in AFs level [95].

4. From lab bench to field trials

Hundreds of BCAs have been tested against different types and strains of mycotoxigenic fungi *in vitro*. However, not all of them were effective against mycotoxigenic fungi under field conditions. For instance, Johansson et al. selected 164 bacterial isolates out of 600 for a field experiment to control *F. culmorum* infection in wheat and three strains of *Fluorescent pseudomonads* and a species of *Pantoea* gave a high level of control and consistent results [159].

In general, the difference in BCAs performance from *in vivo* condition to field conditions might be related to the influence of other factors present in the field such as meteorological parameters, soil characteristics, nutrient availability, microbial community which may affect the efficacy of the screened BCAs. Other important parameters which are not present in *in vivo* studies include the way of delivery of the BCAs to the host (spray or direct inoculation), form of delivery (conidial or spore suspension/with or without carrier), application time (during seeding or flowering) and application route (to the soil or directly to the seed) to ensure the interaction of BCAs against the pathogen. Examples for the available BCAs in the market include AF36 and Afla-Guard® which are commercial BCAs for pre-harvest application to control aflatoxin contamination in the United States [62], Polyversum®, a recent authorized commercial product in France (Pythium oligandrum strain ATCC 38472) to be used against *Alternaria* spp., *Fusarium* spp., and other plant pathogens, and Plant ShieldTM which is the registered product for *T. harzianum* 22.

It is crucial to test all the application related parameters in the field as these parameters may give significantly variable results which are not usually followed in many of the performed field trials against mycotoxigenic caused diseases. For example, point inoculation of *Streptomyces sp.* BN1 was not effective to control FHB in wheat while spraying of bacterial spores during wheat flowering gives better results [175]. Successful formulation of *C. rosea* ACM941 guaranteed its efficacy to control FHB in corn, soybean and wheat under filed conditions [176], while most of the field trials used a conidial or spore suspension of the BCAs which may give variable and inconsistent results. Ear inoculation with *B. amyloliquefaciens* and *Enterobacter hormaechei* exhibit highly changeable results while treatment of seeds showed more stable results for managing *F. verticillioides* infection and toxin content in maize [150]. On the other hand, *B. subtilis* strains SB01, SB04, SB23, and SB24 were performing better to control root rot disease when they were applied to soil than treatment of soybean seeds [145]. Omitting one or more of the above parameters may lead to misevaluation of the selected BCAs.

In some cases, a mixture of two more BCAs maybe advisable in the field for a better disease control in case they have a synergistic effect. For example, mixture of *L. plantarum* SLG17 and *B. amyloliquefaciens* FLN13 showed more efficacy in controlling FHB in wheat durum [131].

Although the field trials are exhausting and time consuming, it should consider the application way, application time, effective dose and the best formula in order to precisely evaluate the performance of the selected BCAs and thereafter ensure an effective control of the mycotoxigenic fungal infection and their mycotoxins.

An important obstacle in the commercialization of BCAs is legislation. Current legislations in Europe classify BCAs as Plant Protection Products/Pesticides and hence they must follow the according regulations of the pesticides. This entails that for each BCA the mode of action must be documented and their use should be rational [177].

5. Conclusions and future perspectives

Despite the considerable amount of research that have been done to screen and select effective BCAs to control mycotoxigenic pathogens and their mycotoxins, still there are several pitfalls for using BCAs. For instance, the broad spectrum antagonistic activity of some BCAs such as *Trichoderma* spp., against several pathogenic fungi may also affect other beneficial organisms present in rhizosphere [178] and this may require more research for target specific BCAs. Even though implementation of a biological control strategy is strongly recommended to replace the use of synthetic pesticides, there are several concerns regarding the biological and environmental stability of BCAs. For example, the population of *A. flavus* including atoxigenic strains is highly diverse. This entails that there is a risk under certain environmental conditions that atoxigenic strains outcross with toxigenic *A. flavus* and thereafter produce mycotoxins [26, 62]. In addition, it is not guaranteed whether the atoxigenic strains can survive for a long time and what is the short term and long term effect on the soil microenvironment.

Care should be taken that besides successful control of plant pathogens, and BCAs themselves do not produce toxic substances. For instance, *C. rosea* secretes gliotoxin which is toxic metabolite to human. Also, it was reported that some *Trichoderma* strains harbor trichothecenes (*Tri*) genes that translate into proteins similar to *Fusarium* Tri proteins [179, 180]. This entails that *Trichoderma* spp. share the production of trichothecenes toxins (such as T-2 toxin) with *Fusarium* spp. In addition, gliotoxin and viridian produced by *T. harzianum*, *T. viride* and *T. virens* showed their phytotoxic effect by reducing seed germination rate in wheat and human toxicity [28]. Therefore, spreading such a microorganism into the environment may impose an extra burden to food safety and public health. Additionally, from the economical point of view, it is necessary to estimate the total cost of application and the need for seasonal reapplication of the BCAs, so it does not exceed costs of current practices.

Controlling mycotoxins is an important aspect in the management of mycotoxigenic pathogens, which adds an extra challenge to find an effective biocontrol agent to control the fungal growth and toxin production simultaneously. It is very well known that one fungal pathogen can produce simultaneously several unrelated mycotoxins, as an example *F. graminearum* produces DON and ZEN which both have two different biosynthetic pathways. The scientific research has mostly been focusing to control one type of mycotoxin. Consequently, it will be more valuable to select a single biocontrol agent able to simultaneously suppress the production of both toxins. It is crucial that the selected BCAs are tolerant to mycotoxins [169] which will guarantee the long term efficiency in the field.

Some mycotoxins can be modified by the plant through alteration of their chemical structure "i.e. conjugation to a glucose moiety and hence called plant metabolites of mycotoxins or modified or masked mycotoxins" [181]. For example, DON is transformed to deoxynivalenol-3-glucoside (DON3G) in the plant as a part of the plant defense mechanism. These masked forms of mycotoxins can be hydrolyzed back into their parent forms "DON" inside human and animal body. Therefore, it is of paramount importance to take into account the effect of biocontrol agents on the production of (masked) mycotoxins and to deeply investigate whether the efficacy of the selected BCAs is due to an actual reduction of mycotoxin content based on a direct inhibition of their production by the pathogen or due to enhancing the plant immunity which may increase the plant ability to form more DON3G as in this case the total mycotoxin content in the plant will remain unchanged. Furthermore, the underlying mechanism between the parent mycotoxin, host and BCAs remains obscure and should be further investigated. In addition, other categories of mycotoxins, however they pose health risks, are underexplored such as enniatins, emerging mycotoxins produced by *Fusarium* spp., [14, 182] have not been tested with BCAs and this necessitates the need for further investigation.

Different BCAs with different modes of action, formulation, treatments, application time were tested showing that it may be difficult to have a single BCA able to diminish all the regulated mycotoxins "one fits for all may not be the case here" [183, 184]. To tackle this problem, maybe a combination of multiple BCAs or with fungicides could be considered. Application dose should be deeply investigated to achieve the desirable control. As in previous research, it has been shown that a suboptimal or sublethal treatment with fungicides [185] may lead to induction of mycotoxins production by the pathogen as a stress response. Searching for new BCAs with novel modes of action can assist to effectively control mycotoxigenic plant pathogens. Recently, *Enterobacter* spp., a root-inhabiting bacterial endophyte, was reported to have a different mode of action than those previously described through formation of physicochemical barrier that blocks the invasion of *F. graminearum*. However it is unclear whether this mode of action can be applied to maize and wheat [186]. Finally, the sound implantation of pre-harvest strategies can help in saving crop loss but does not fully ensure the safety of food as the fungal attack can also happen during storage or during processing which necessitate a post-harvest control.

Acknowledgements

This work was supported by the EU project Horizon 2020-MYCOKEY "Integrated and innovative key actions for mycotoxin management in the food".

Conflict of interest

The authors declare no conflict of interest.

Other declarations

The authors have mentioned some trade names of certain BCAs for the scientific purpose only and this does not reflect any recommendation for use.

Author details

Mohamed F. Abdallah[1,2*], Maarten Ameye[1], Sarah De Saeger[2], Kris Audenaert[1] and Geert Haesaert[1*]

*Address all correspondence to: mohamed.fathi@ugent.be; geert.haesaert@ugent.be

1 Laboratory of Applied Mycology and Phenomics, Department of Plants and Crops, Faculty of Bioscience Engineering, Ghent University, Ghent, Belgium

2 Centre of Excellence in Mycotoxicology and Public Health, Department of Bioanalysis, Faculty of Pharmaceutical Sciences, Ghent University, Ghent, Belgium

References

[1] FAO. How to Feed the World in 2050. 2009. Available from http://www.fao.org/fileadmin/templates/wsfs/docs/expert_paper/How_to_Feed_the_World_in_2050.pdf [Accessed: January 5, 2018]

[2] Sasson A. Food security for Africa: An urgent global challenge. Agricultural Food Security. 2012;**1**(2)

[3] Fisher MC, Henk DA, Briggs CJ, et al. Emerging fungal threats to animal, plant and ecosystem health. Nature. 2012;**484**:186-194

[4] Bennett JW, Klich M, Mycotoxins M. Mycotoxins. Clinical Microbiology Review. 2003;**16**: 497-516

[5] Zain ME. Impact of mycotoxins on humans and animals. Journal of Saudi Chemical Society. 2011;**15**:129-144

[6] De Ruyck K, De Boevre M, Huybrechts I, et al. Dietary mycotoxins, co-exposure, and carcinogenesis in humans: Short review. Mutation Research, Reviews in Mutation Research. 2015;**766**:32-41

[7] Pal KK, Mc Spadden Gardener B. Biological control of plant pathogens. Plant Heal Instructor. 2006:1-25

[8] Weller DM. Biological control of soilborne plant pathogens in the rhizosphere with bacteria. Annual Review of Phytopathology. 1988;**26**:379-407

[9] Agrios GN. Control of plant diseases. Plant Pathology. 1969;**28**:173-206

[10] El-Tarabily KA, Sivasithamparam K. Potential of yeasts as biocontrol agents of soil-borne fungal plant pathogens and as plant growth promoters. Mycoscience. 2006;**47**:25-35

[11] Punja ZK, Utkhede RS. Using fungi and yeasts to manage vegetable crop diseases. Trends in Biotechnology. 2003;**21**:400-407

[12] Droby S, Wisniewski M, Macarisin D, et al. Twenty years of postharvest biocontrol research: Is it time for a new paradigm? Postharvest Biology and Technology. 2009;**52**: 137-145

[13] Torres AM, Barros GG, Palacios SA, et al. Review on pre- and post-harvest management of peanuts to minimize aflatoxin contamination. Food Research International. 2014;**62**: 11-19

[14] Ferrigo D, Raiola A, Causin R. Fusarium toxins in cereals: Occurrence, legislation, factors promoting the appearance and their management. Molecules. 2016;**21**:627

[15] Yazar S, Omurtag GZ. Fumonisins, trichothecenes and zearalenone in cereals. International Journal of Molecular Sciences. 2008;**9**:2062-2090

[16] Pitt JI, Miller JD. A concise history of Mycotoxin research. Journal of Agricultural and Food Chemistry. DOI: 10.1021/acs.jafc.6b04494

[17] Marin S, Ramos AJJ, Cano-Sancho G, et al. Mycotoxins: Occurrence, toxicology, and exposure assessment. Food and Chemical Toxicology. 2013;**60**:218-237

[18] Voss KA, Smith GW, Haschek WM. Fumonisins: Toxicokinetics, mechanism of action and toxicity. Animal Feed Science and Technology. 2007;**137**:299-325

[19] Wang J, Liu J, Chen H, et al. Characterization of *Fusarium graminearum* inhibitory lipopeptide from Bacillus subtilis IB. Applied Microbiology and Biotechnology. 2007;**76**: 889-894

[20] Nagórska K, Bikowski M, Obuchowski M. Multicellular behaviour and production of a wide variety of toxic substances support usage of Bacillus subtilis as a powerful biocontrol agent. Acta Biochimica Polonica. 2007;**54**:495-508

[21] Couillerot O, Prigent-Combaret C, Caballero-Mellado J, et al. Pseudomonas fluorescens and closely-related fluorescent pseudomonads as biocontrol agents of soil-borne phytopathogens. Letters in Applied Microbiology. 2009;**48**:505-512

[22] El-Tarabily KA, Sivasithamparam K. Non-streptomycete actinomycetes as biocontrol agents of soil-borne fungal plant pathogens and as plant growth promoters. Soil Biology and Biochemistry. 2006;**38**:1505-1520

[23] Daguerre Y, Siegel K, Edel-Hermann V, et al. Fungal proteins and genes associated with biocontrol mechanisms of soil-borne pathogens: A review. Fungal Biology Reviews. 2014;**28**:97-125

[24] Benítez T, Rincón AM, Limón MC, et al. Biocontrol mechanisms of Trichoderma strains. International Microbiology. 2004;**7**:249-260

[25] Alabouvette C, Olivain C, Migheli Q, et al. Microbiological control of soil-borne phytopathogenic fungi with special emphasis on wilt-inducing Fusarium oxysporum. The New Phytologist. 2009;**184**:529-544

[26] Ehrlich KC. Non-aflatoxigenic *Aspergillus flavus* to prevent aflatoxin contamination in crops: Advantages and limitations. Frontiers in Microbiology. 2014;**5**:1-9

[27] Abbas H, Zablotowicz R, Bruns HA, et al. Biocontrol of aflatoxin in corn by inoculation with non-aflatoxigenic *Aspergillus flavus* isolates. Biocontrol Science and Technology. 2006;**16**:437-449

[28] Kim SH, Vujanovic V. Relationship between mycoparasites lifestyles and biocontrol behaviors against Fusarium spp. and mycotoxins production. Applied Microbiology and Biotechnology. 2016;**100**:5257-5272

[29] Howell CR. Mechanisms employed by Trichoderma species in the biological control of plant diseases: The history and evolution of current concepts. Plant Disease. 2003;**87**:4-10

[30] Barnett HL. The nature of Mycoparasitism by Fungi. Annual Review of Microbiology. 1963;**17**:1-14

[31] Shoresh M, Harman GE, Mastouri F. Induced systemic resistance and plant responses to fungal biocontrol agents. Annual Review of Phytopathology. 2010;**48**:21-43

[32] Lugtenberg BJJ, Caradus JR, Johnson LJ. Fungal endophytes for sustainable crop production. FEMS Microbiology Ecology. 2016;**92**:1-17

[33] Xue AG, Voldeng HD, Savard ME, et al. Biological control of fusarium head blight of wheat with Clonostachys rosea strain ACM941. Canadian Journal of Plant Pathology. 2009;**31**:169-179

[34] Gupta CP, Dubey RC, Kang SC, et al. Antibiosis-mediated necrotrophic effect of Pseudomonas GRC 2 against two fungal plant pathogens. Current Science. 2001;**81**:91-94

[35] Zhao Y, Selvaraj JN, Xing F, et al. Antagonistic action of Bacillus subtilis strain SG6 on *Fusarium graminearum*. PLoS One. 2014;**9**:1-11

[36] Etcheverry MG, Scandolara A, Nesci A, et al. Biological interactions to select biocontrol agents against toxigenic strains of *Aspergillus flavus* and fusarium verticillioides from maize. Mycopathologia. 2009;**167**:287-295

[37] Vinale F, Sivasithamparam K, Ghisalberti EL, et al. Trichoderma-plant-pathogen interactions. Soil Biology and Biochemistry. 2008;**40**:1-10

[38] Calistru C, McLean M, Berjak P. In vitro studies on the potential for biological control of *Aspergillus flavus* and Fusarium moniliforme by Trichoderma species. A study of the production of extracellular metabolites by Trichoderma species. Mycopathologia. 1997; **137**:115-124

[39] Romero D, de Vicente A, Rakotoaly RH, et al. The Iturin and Fengycin families of Lipopeptides are key factors in antagonism of Bacillus subtilis toward Podosphaera fusca. Molecular Plant-Microbe Interactions 2007;**20**:430-440

[40] Veras FF, Correa APF, Welke JE, et al. Inhibition of mycotoxin-producing fungi by Bacillus strains isolated from fish intestines. International Journal of Food Microbiology. 2016;**238**:23-32

[41] Mohammadipour M, Mousivand M, Salehi Jouzani G, et al. Molecular and biochemical characterization of Iranian surfactin-producing Bacillus subtilis isolates and evaluation of their biocontrol potential against *Aspergillus flavus* and Colletotrichum gloeosporioides. Canadian Journal of Microbiology. 2009;**55**:395-404

[42] Crane JM, Gibson DM, Vaughan RH, et al. Iturin levels on wheat spikes linked to biological control of Fusarium head blight by Bacillus amyloliquefaciens. Phytopathology. 2013;**103**:146-155

[43] Maurhofer M, Baehler E, Notz R, et al. Cross talk between 2,4-Diacetylphloroglucinol-producing biocontrol pseudomonads on wheat roots. Applied and Environmental Microbiology. 2004;**70**:1990-1998

[44] Mavrodi OV, McSpadden Gardener BB, Mavrodi DV, et al. Genetic diversity of phlD from 2,4-Diacetylphloroglucinol-producing fluorescent Pseudomonas spp. Phytopathology. 2001;**91**:35-43

[45] Brazelton JN, Pfeufer EE, Sweat TA, et al. 2,4-Diacetylphloroglucinol alters plant root development. Molecular Plant-Microbe Interactions. 2008;**21**:1349-1358

[46] Shanahan P, O'Sullivan DJ, Simpson P, et al. Isolation of 2,4-diacetylphloroglucinol from a fluorescent pseudomonad and investigation of physiological parameters influencing its production. Applied and Environmental Microbiology. 1992;**58**:353-358

[47] De La Fuente L, Mavrodi DV, Landa BB, et al. phlD-based genetic diversity and detection of genotypes of 2,4- diacetylphloroglucinol-producing Pseudomonas fluorescens. FEMS Microbiology Ecology. 2006;**56**:64-78

[48] Müller T, Behrendt U, Ruppel S, et al. Fluorescent pseudomonads in the Phyllosphere of wheat: Potential antagonists against fungal Phytopathogens. Current Microbiology. 2016;**72**:383-389

[49] Gao M, Glenn AE, Blacutt AA, et al. Fungal lactamases: Their occurrence and function. Frontiers in Microbiology. 2017;**8**:1775

[50] Lakhesar DPS, Backhouse D, Kristiansen P. Nutritional constraints on displacement of Fusarium pseudograminearum from cereal straw by antagonists. Biological Control. 2010;**55**:241-247

[51] Dawson WAJM, Jestoi M, Rizzo A, et al. Field evaluation of fungal competitors of Fusarium culmorum and F. Graminearum, causal agents of ear blight of winter wheat, for the control of Mycotoxin production in grain. Biocontrol Science and Technology. 2004;**14**:783-799

[52] Cotty PJ. Virulence and cultural characteristics of two *Aspergillus flavus* strains pathogenic on cotton. Phytopathology. 1989;**79**:808-814

[53] Cotty PJ, Bhatnagar D. Variability among atoxigenic *Aspergillus flavus* strains in ability to prevent aflatoxin contamination and production of aflatoxin biosynthetic pathway enzymes. Applied and Environmental Microbiology. 1994;**60**:2248-2251

[54] Cotty PJ. Effect of Atoxigenic strains of *Aspergillus flavus* on Aflatoxin contamination of developing cottonseed. Plant Disease. 1990;**74**:233-235

[55] Atehnkeng J, Ojiambo PS, Cotty PJ, et al. Field efficacy of a mixture of atoxigenic *Aspergillus flavus* link: FR vegetative compatibility groups in preventing aflatoxin contamination in maize (Zea mays L.). Biological Control. 2014;**72**:62-70

[56] Dorner JW. Biological control of aflatoxin contamination in corn using a nontoxigenic strain of *Aspergillus flavus*. Journal of Food Protection. 2009;**72**:801-804

[57] Dorner JW. Efficacy of a biopesticide for control of aflatoxins in corn. Journal of Food Protection. 2010;**73**:495-499

[58] Alaniz Zanon MS, Barros GG, Chulze SN. Non-aflatoxigenic *Aspergillus flavus* as potential biocontrol agents to reduce aflatoxin contamination in peanuts harvested in northern Argentina. International Journal of Food Microbiology. 2016;**231**:63-68

[59] Alaniz Zanon MS, Chiotta ML, Giaj-Merlera G, et al. Evaluation of potential biocontrol agent for aflatoxin in Argentinean peanuts. International Journal of Food Microbiology. 2013;**162**:220-225

[60] Horn BW, Dorner JW. Effect of nontoxigenic *Aspergillus flavus* and *A. parasiticus* on aflatoxin contamination of wounded peanut seeds inoculated with agricultural soil containing natural fungal populations. Biocontrol Science and Technology. 2009;**19**:249-262

[61] Hulikunte Mallikarjunaiah N, Jayapala N, Puttaswamy H, et al. Characterization of non-aflatoxigenic strains of *Aspergillus flavus* as potential biocontrol agent for the management of aflatoxin contamination in groundnut. Microbial Pathogenesis. 2017;**102**:21-28

[62] Hruska Z, Rajasekaran K, Yao H, et al. Co-inoculation of aflatoxigenic and non-aflatoxigenic strains of *Aspergillus flavus* to study fungal invasion, colonization, and competition in maize kernels. Frontiers in Microbiology. 2014;**5**:122. DOI: 10.3389/fmicb.2014.00122

[63] Chang P-K, Ehrlich KC. Cyclopiazonic acid biosynthesis by *Aspergillus flavus*. Toxin Reviews. 2011;**30**:79-89

[64] Uka V, Moore GG, Arroyo-Manzanares N, et al. Unravelling the diversity of the cyclopiazonic acid family of mycotoxins in *Aspergillus flavus* by UHPLC triple-TOF HRMS. Toxins. 2017;**9**:35. DOI: 10.3390/toxins9010035

[65] Abbas HK, Zablotowicz RM, Horn BW, et al. Comparison of major biocontrol strains of non-aflatoxigenic *Aspergillus flavus* for the reduction of aflatoxins and cyclopiazonic acid in maize. Food Addit Contam - Part A Chem Anal Control Expo Risk Assess. 2011;**28**: 198-208

[66] Zhou L, Wei D, Selvaraj JN, et al. A strain of *Aspergillus flavus* from China shows potential as a biocontrol agent for aflatoxin contamination. Biocontrol Science and Technology. 2015;**25**:583-592

[67] Mauro A, Battilani P, Cotty PJ. Atoxigenic *Aspergillus flavus* endemic to Italy for biocontrol of aflatoxins in maize. BioControl. 2015;**60**:125-134

[68] Verma M, Brar SK, Tyagi RD, et al. Antagonistic fungi, Trichoderma spp.: Panoply of biological control. Biochemical Engineering Journal. 2007;**37**:1-20

[69] Altomare C, Norvell WA, Björkman T, et al. Solubilization of phosphates and micronutrients by the plant-growth- promoting and biocontrol fungus Trichoderma harzianum Rifai 1295-22. Applied and Environmental Microbiology. 1999;**65**:2926-2933

[70] Harman GE, Howell CR, Viterbo A, et al. Trichoderma species - opportunistic, avirulent plant symbionts. Nature Reviews. Microbiology. 2004;**2**:43-56

[71] Druzhinina IS, Seidl-Seiboth V, Herrera-Estrella A, et al. Trichoderma: The genomics of opportunistic success. Nature Reviews. Microbiology. 2011;**9**:749-759

[72] Matarese F, Sarrocco S, Gruber S, et al. Biocontrol of Fusarium head blight: Interactions between Trichoderma and mycotoxigenic Fusarium. Microbiology. 2012;**158**:98-106

[73] Yates IE, Meredith F, Smart W, et al. Trichoderma viride suppresses fumonisin B1 production by *Fusarium moniliforme*. Journal of Food Protection. 1999;**62**:1326-1332

[74] Sempere F, Santamarina MP. Antagonistic interactions between fungal rice pathogen *Fusarium verticillioides* (Sacc.) Nirenberg and *Trichoderma harzianum* Rifai. Annales de Microbiologie. 2009;**59**:259-266

[75] Sempere F, Santamarina MP. In vitro biocontrol analysis of Alternaria alternata (Fr.) Keissler under different environmental conditions. Mycopathologia. 2007;**163**:183-190

[76] Dal Bello GM, Mónaco CI, Simón MR. Biological control of seedling bright of wheat caused by *Fusarium graminearum* with beneficial rhizosphere microorganisms. World Journal of Microbiology and Biotechnology. 2002;**18**:627-636

[77] Inch S, Gilbert J. Effect of *Trichoderma harzianum* on perithecial production of Gibberella zeae on wheat straw. Biocontrol Science and Technology. 2007;**17**:635-646

[78] Schoneberg A, Musa T, Voegele RT, et al. The potential of antagonistic fungi for control of *Fusarium graminearum* and *Fusarium crookwellense* varies depending on the experimental approach. Journal of Applied Microbiology. 2015;**118**:1165-1179

[79] Roberti R, Veronesi AR, Cesari A, et al. Induction of PR proteins and resistance by the biocontrol agent *Clonostachys rosea* in wheat plants infected with *Fusarium culmorum*. Plant Science. 2008;**175**:339-347

[80] Samsudin NIP, Medina A, Magan N. Relationship between environmental conditions, carbon utilisation patterns and niche overlap indices of the mycotoxigenic species *Fusarium verticillioides* and the biocontrol agent *Clonostachys rosea*. Fungal Ecology. 2016;**24**:44-52

[81] Mamarabadi M, Jensen DF, Lübeck M. An N-acetyl-β-d-glucosaminidase gene, cr-nag1, from the biocontrol agent *Clonostachys rosea* is up-regulated in antagonistic interactions with *Fusarium culmorum*. Mycological Research. 2009;**113**:33-43

[82] Vujanovic V, Goh YK. Sphaerodes mycoparasitica sp. nov., a new biotrophic mycoparasite on *Fusarium avenaceum*, *F. graminearum* and *F. oxysporum*. Mycological Research. 2009;**113**:1172-1180

[83] Vujanovic V, Goh YK. Qpcr quantification of sphaerodes mycoparasitica biotrophic mycoparasite interaction with *Fusarium graminearum*: In vitro and in planta assays. Archives of Microbiology. 2012;**194**:707-717

[84] Palumbo JD, O'Keeffe TL, Abbas HK. Isolation of maize soil and rhizosphere bacteria with antagonistic activity against *Aspergillus flavus* and *Fusarium verticillioides*. Journal of Food Protection. 2007;**70**:1615-1621

[85] Heil M, Bostock RM. Induced systemic resistance (ISR) against pathogens in the context of induced plant defences. Annals of Botany. 2002;**89**:503-512

[86] Choudhary DK, Prakash A, Johri BN. Induced systemic resistance (ISR) in plants: Mechanism of action. Indian Journal of Microbiology. 2007;**47**:289-297

[87] Pieterse CMJ, Zamioudis C, Berendsen RL, et al. Induced systemic resistance by beneficial microbes. Annual Review of Phytopathology. 2014;**52**:347-375

[88] Mantelin S, Touraine B. Plant growth-promoting bacteria and nitrate availability: Impacts on root development and nitrate uptake. Journal of Experimental Botany. 2004; **55**:27-34

[89] Alimi M, Javad M, Darzi MT. Characterization and application of microbial antagonists for control of Fusarium head blight of wheat caused by *Fusarium graminearum* using single and mixture strain of antagonistic bacteria on resistance and susceptible cultivars. African Journal of Microbiological Research. 2012;**6**:326-334

[90] Hernández-Rodríguez A, Heydrich-Pérez M, Acebo-Guerrero Y, et al. Antagonistic activity of Cuban native rhizobacteria against *Fusarium verticillioides* (Sacc.) Nirenb. In maize (*Zea mays* L.). Applied Soil Ecology. 2008;**39**:180-186

[91] Henkes GJ, Jousset A, Bonkowski M, et al. *Pseudomonas fluorescens* CHA0 maintains carbon delivery to *Fusarium graminearum*-infected roots and prevents reduction in biomass of barley shoots through systemic interactions. Journal of Experimental Botany. 2011;**62**:4337-4344

[92] Khan MR, Fischer S, Egan D, et al. Biological control of Fusarium seedling blight disease of wheat and barley. Phytopathology. 2006;**69**:386-394

[93] Jochum CC, Osborne LE, Yuen GY. Fusarium head blight biological control with Lysobacter enzymogenes strain C3. Biological Control. 2006;**39**:336-344

[94] Danielsen S, Funck Jensen D. Fungal endophytes from stalks of tropical maize and grasses: Isolation, identification, and screening for antagonism against *Fusarium verticillioides* in maize stalks. Biocontrol Science and Technology. 1999;**9**:545-553

[95] Aiyaz M, Divakara ST, Nayaka SC, et al. Application of beneficial rhizospheric microbes for the mitigation of seed-borne mycotoxigenic fungal infection and mycotoxins in maize. Biocontrol Science and Technology. 2015;**25**:1105-1119

[96] Ferrigo D, Raiola A, Piccolo E, et al. Trichoderma harzianum T22 induces in maize systemic resistance against *Fusarium verticillioides*. Journal of Plant Pathology. 2014;**96**: 133-142

[97] Mukherjee M, Mukherjee PK, Horwitz BA, et al. Trichoderma-plant-pathogen interactions: Advances in genetics of biological control. Indian Journal of Microbiology. 2012;**52**: 522-529

[98] Porras-Alfaro A, Bayman P. Hidden fungi, emergent properties: Endophytes and microbiomes. Annual Review of Phytopathology. 2011;**49**:291-315

[99] Mousa WK, Shearer CR, Limay-Rios V, et al. Bacterial endophytes from wild maize suppress *Fusarium graminearum* in modern maize and inhibit mycotoxin accumulation. Frontiers in Plant Science. 2015;**6**:805

[100] Rabiey M, Shaw MW. *Piriformospora indica* reduces fusarium head blight disease severity and mycotoxin DON contamination in wheat under UK weather conditions. Plant Pathology. 2016;**65**:940-952

[101] Rabiey M, Ullah I, Shaw MW. The endophytic fungus *Piriformospora indica* protects wheat from fusarium crown rot disease in simulated UK autumn conditions. Plant Pathology. 2015;**64**:1029-1040

[102] Waller F, Achatz B, Baltruschat H, et al. The endophytic fungus *Piriformospora indica* reprograms barley to salt-stress tolerance, disease resistance, and higher yield. Proceedings of the National Academy of Sciences. 2005;**102**:13386-13391

[103] Deshmukh SD, Kogel K-H. *Piriformospora indica* protects barley from root rot caused by *Fusarium graminearum*. Journal of Plant Disease Protocol. 2007;**114**:263-268

[104] Varma A, Verma S, Sudha, et al. Piriformospora indica, a cultivable plant-growth-promoting root endophyte. Applied and Environmental Microbiology. 1999;**65**:2741-2744

[105] Sherameti I, Shahollari B, Venus Y, et al. The endophytic fungus *Piriformospora indica* stimulates the expression of nitrate reductase and the starch-degrading enzyme glucan-water dikinase in tobacco and Arabidopsis roots through a homeodomain transcription factor that binds to a conserved motif in. The Journal of Biological Chemistry. 2005;**280**: 26241-26247

[106] Ogórek R, Plaskowska E. *Epicoccum nigrum* for biocontrol agents in vitro of plant fungal pathogens. Communications in Agricultural and Applied Biological Sciences. 2011;**76**: 691-697

[107] Musyimi SL, Muthomi JW, Narla RD, et al. Efficacy of biological control and cultivar resistance on Fusarium head blight and T-2 toxin contamination in wheat. American Journal of Plant Sciences. 2012;**3**:599-607

[108] Jensen BD, Knorr K, Nicolaisen M. In vitro competition between *Fusarium graminearum* and *Epicoccum nigrum* on media and wheat grains. European Journal of Plant Pathology. 2016;**146**:657-670

[109] Sempere F, Saiilamarina MP. Study of the interactions between *Penicillium oxalicum* Currie & thom and Alternaria alternata (fr.) keissler. Brazilian Journal of Microbiology. 2010;**41**:700-706

[110] Ammar HAM, Awny NM, Fahmy HM. Influence of environmental conditions of atoxigenic *Aspergillus flavus* HFB1 on biocontrol of patulin produced by a novel apple

contaminant isolate, A. terreusHAP1, in vivo and in vitro. Biocatalysis and Agricultural Biotechnology. 2017;**12**:36-44

[111] Bleve G, Grieco F, Cozzi G, et al. Isolation of epiphytic yeasts with potential for biocontrol of *Aspergillus carbonarius* and *A. niger* on grape. International Journal of Food Microbiology. 2006;**108**:204-209

[112] Dimakopoulou M, Tjamos SE, Antoniou PP, et al. Phyllosphere grapevine yeast *Aureobasidium pullulans* reduces *Aspergillus carbonarius* (sour rot) incidence in wine-producing vineyards in Greece. Biological Control. 2008;**46**:158-165

[113] Afsharmanesh H, Ahmadzadeh M, Javan-Nikkhah M, et al. Improvement in biocontrol activity of Bacillus subtilis UTB1 against *Aspergillus flavus* using gamma-irradiation. Crop Protection. 2014;**60**:83-92

[114] Doster MA, Cotty PJ, Michailides TJ. Evaluation of the Atoxigenic *Aspergillus flavus* strain AF36 in pistachio orchards. Plant Disease. 2014;**98**:948-956

[115] Anjaiah V, Thakur RP, Koedam N. Evaluation of bacteria and Trichoderma for biocontrol of pre-harvest seed infection by *Aspergillus flavus* in groundnut. Biocontrol Science and Technology. 2006;**16**:431-436

[116] Desai S, Thakur RP, Rao VP, et al. Characterization of isolates of Trichoderma for biocontrol potential against *Aspergillus flavus* infection in groundnut. International Arachis Newsletter. 2000:57-59

[117] Sultan Y, Magan N. Impact of a Streptomyces (AS1) strain and its metabolites on control of *Aspergillus flavus* and aflatoxin B1contamination in vitro and in stored peanuts. Biocontrol Science and Technology. 2011;**21**:1437-1455

[118] Gong AD, Li HP, Shen L, et al. The Shewanella algae strain YM8 produces volatiles with strong inhibition activity against Aspergillus pathogens and aflatoxins. Frontiers in Microbiology. 2015;**6**:1-12

[119] Dorner JW, Horn BW. Separate and combined applications of nontoxigenic *Aspergillus flavus* and *A. parasiticus* for biocontrol of aflatoxin in peanuts. Mycopathologia. 2007;**163**: 215-223

[120] Atehnkeng J, Ojiambo PS, Ikotun T, et al. Evaluation of atoxigenic isolates of *Aspergillus flavus* as potential biocontrol agents for aflatoxin in maize. Food Addition Contamination - Part A Chemical Analysis Control Expo Risk Assess. 2008;**25**:1264-1271

[121] Nesci AV, Bluma RV, Etcheverry MG. In vitro selection of maize rhizobacteria to study potential biological control of Aspergillus section Flavi and aflatoxin production. European Journal of Plant Pathology. 2005;**113**:159-171

[122] Degola F, Berni E, Restivo FM. Laboratory tests for assessing efficacy of atoxigenic *Aspergillus flavus* strains as biocontrol agents. International Journal of Food Microbiology. 2011;**146**:235-243

[123] Probst C, Bandyopadhyay R, Price LE, et al. Identification of Atoxigenic *Aspergillus flavus* isolates to reduce Aflatoxin contamination of maize in Kenya. Plant Disease. 2011;**95**: 212-218

[124] Al-Saad LA, Al-Badran AI, Al-Jumayli SA, et al. Impact of bacterial biocontrol agents on aflatoxin biosynthetic genes, aflD and aflR expression, and phenotypic aflatoxin B1 production by *Aspergillus flavus* under different environmental and nutritional regimes. International Journal of Food Microbiology. 2016;**217**:123-129

[125] Sailaja PR, Podile AR, Reddanna P. Biocontrol strain of Bacillus subtilis AF 1 rapidly induces lipoxygenase in groundnut (*Arachis hypogaea* L.) compared to crown rot pathogen *Aspergillus niger*. European Journal of Plant Pathology. 1998;**104**:125-132

[126] Nagaraja H, Chennappa G, Rakesh S, et al. Antifungal activity of *Azotobacter nigricans* against trichothecene-producing Fusarium species associated with cereals. Food Science and Biotechnology. 2016;**25**:1197-1204

[127] Palazzini JM, Groenenboom-de Haas BH, Torres AM, et al. Biocontrol and population dynamics of fusarium spp. on wheat stubble in Argentina. Plant Pathology. 2013;**62**: 859-866

[128] Gromadzka K, Chelkowski J, Popiel D, et al. Solid substrate bioassay to evaluate the effect of Trichoderma and Clonostachys on the production of zearalenone by Fusarium species. World Mycotoxin Journal. 2009;**2**:45-52

[129] Luongo L, Galli M, Corazza L, et al. Potential of fungal antagonists for biocontrol of Fusarium spp. in wheat and maize through competition in crop debris. Biocontrol Science and Technology. 2005;**15**:229-242

[130] Comby M, Gacoin M, Robineau M, et al. Screening of wheat endophytes as biological control agents against Fusarium head blight using two different in vitro tests. Microbiological Research. 2017;**202**:11-20

[131] Baffoni L, Gaggia F, Dalanaj N, et al. Microbial inoculants for the biocontrol of Fusarium spp. in durum wheat. BMC Microbiology. 2015;**15**:8-10

[132] Wachowska U, Głowacka K. Antagonistic interactions between *Aureobasidium pullulans* and *Fusarium culmorum*, a fungal pathogen of winter wheat. BioControl. 2014;**59**:635-645

[133] Ferre FS, Santamarina MP. Efficacy of trichoderma harzianum in suppression of *Fusarium culmorum*. Annales de Microbiologie. 2010;**60**:335-340

[134] Vujanovic V, Goh YK. Sphaerodes mycoparasitica biotrophic mycoparasite of 3- acetyldeoxynivalenol- and 15-acetyldeoxynivalenol-producing toxigenic *Fusarium graminearum* chemotypes. FEMS Microbiology Letters. 2011;**316**:136-143

[135] Yoshida S, Ohba A, Liang YM, et al. Specificity of Pseudomonas isolates on healthy and Fusarium head blight-infected Spikelets of wheat heads. Microbial Ecology. 2012;**64**: 214-225

[136] Zalila-Kolsi I, Ben Mahmoud A, Ali H, et al. Antagonist effects of *Bacillus* spp. strains against *Fusarium graminearum* for protection of durum wheat (*Triticum turgidum* L. subsp. durum). Microbiological Research. 2016;**192**:148-158

[137] Khan NI, Schisler DA, Boehm MJ, et al. Field testing of antagonists of Fusarium head blight incited by Gibberella zeae. Biological Control. 2004;**29**:245-255

[138] Shi C, Yan P, Li J, et al. Biocontrol of *Fusarium graminearum* growth and deoxynivalenol production in wheat kernels with bacterial antagonists. International Journal of Environmental Research and Public Health. 2014;**11**:1094-1105

[139] Hu W, Gao Q, Hamada MS, et al. Potential of *Pseudomonas chlororaphis* subsp. aurantiaca strain Pcho10 as a biocontrol agent against *Fusarium graminearum*. Phytopathology. 2014; **104**:1289-1297

[140] Goh Kheng Y, Vujanovic V. Biotrophic mycoparasitic interactions between *Sphaerodes mycoparasitica* and phytopathogenic *Fusarium* species. Biocontrol Science and Technology. 2010;**20**:891-902

[141] Crane JM, Bergstrom GC. Spatial distribution and antifungal interactions of a Bacillus biological control agent on wheat surfaces. Biological Control. 2014;**78**:23-32

[142] Schisler DA, Core AB, Boehm MJ, et al. Population dynamics of the Fusarium head blight biocontrol agent *Cryptococcus flavescens* OH 182.9 on wheat anthers and heads. Biological Control. 2014;**70**:17-27

[143] Moussa TAA, Almaghrabi OA, Abdel-Moneim TS. Biological control of the wheat root rot caused by *Fusarium graminearum* using some PGPR strains in Saudi Arabia. The Annals of Applied Biology. 2013;**163**:72-81

[144] Palazzini JM, Alberione E, Torres A, et al. Biological control of *Fusarium graminearum* sensu stricto, causal agent of Fusarium head blight of wheat, using formulated antagonists under field conditions in Argentina. Biological Control. 2016;**94**:56-61

[145] Zhang JX, Xue AG, Tambong JT. Evaluation of seed and soil treatments with novel Bacillus subtilis strains for control of soybean root rot caused by *Fusarium oxysporum* and *F. graminearum*. Plant Disease. 2009;**93**:7

[146] Dalie DKD, Deschamps a M, Atanasova-Penichon V, et al. Potential of *Pediococcus pentosaceus* (L006) isolated from maize leaf to suppress fumonisin-producing fungal growth. Journal of Food Protection. 2010;**73**:1129-1137

[147] Nayaka SC, Udaya Shankar AC, Reddy MS, et al. Control of *Fusarium verticillioides*, cause of ear rot of maize, by *Pseudomonas fluorescens*. Pest Management Science. 2009;**65**:769-775

[148] Pereira P, Nesci A, Etcheverry M. Effects of biocontrol agents on Fusarium verticillioides count and fumonisin content in the maize agroecosystem: Impact on rhizospheric bacterial and fungal groups. Biological Control. 2007;**42**:281-287

[149] Pereira P, Nesci A, Etcheverry MG. Efficacy of bacterial seed treatments for the control of *Fusarium verticillioides* in maize. BioControl. 2009;**54**:103-111

[150] Pereira P, Nesci A, Castillo C, et al. Impact of bacterial biological control agents on fumonisin B1 content and *Fusarium verticillioides* infection of field-grown maize. Biological Control. 2010;**53**:258-266

[151] Cavaglieri L, Orlando J, Etcheverry M. In vitro influence of bacterial mixtures on Fusarium verticillioides growth and fumonisin B1 production: Effect of seeds treatment on maize root colonization. Letters in Applied Microbiology. 2005;**41**:390-396

[152] Cavaglieri L, Orlando J, Rodríguez MI, et al. Biocontrol of *Bacillus subtilis* against *Fusarium verticillioides* in vitro and at the maize root level. Research in Microbiology. 2005;**156**: 748-754

[153] Figueroa-López AM, Cordero-Ramírez JD, Martínez-Álvarez JC, et al. Rhizospheric bacteria of maize with potential for biocontrol of *Fusarium verticillioides*. Springerplus. DOI: 10.1186/s40064-016-1780-x

[154] Bacon CW, Yates IE, Hinton DM, et al. Biological control of *Fusarium moniliforme* in maize. Environmental Health Perspectives. 2001;**109**:325-332

[155] Samsudin NIP, Magan N. Efficacy of potential biocontrol agents for control of Fusarium verticillioides and fumonisin B 1 under different environmental conditions. World Mycotoxin Journal. 2016;**9**:205-213

[156] Samsudin NIP, Rodriguez A, Medina A, et al. Efficacy of fungal and bacterial antagonists for controlling growth, FUM1 gene expression and fumonisin B1production by *Fusarium verticillioides* on maize cobs of different ripening stages. International Journal of Food Microbiology. 2017;**246**:72-79

[157] Cavaglieri L, Passone A, Etcheverry M. Screening procedures for selecting rhizobacteria with biocontrol effects upon Fusarium verticillioides growth and fumonisin B1 production. Research in Microbiology. 2004;**155**:747-754

[158] Pereira P, Nesci A, Castillo C, et al. Field studies on the relationship between Fusarium verticillioides and maize (*Zea mays* L.): Effect of biocontrol agents on fungal infection and toxin content of grains at harvest. International Journal of Agronomics. 2011;**2011**:1-7

[159] Johansson PM, Johnsson L, Gerhardson B. Suppression of wheat-seedling diseases caused by Fusarium culmorum and Microdochium nivale using bacterial seed treatment. Plant Pathology. 2003;**52**:219-227

[160] Audenaert K, Vanheule A, Höfte M, et al. Deoxynivalenol: A major player in the multifaceted response of Fusarium to its environment. Toxins. 2013;**6**:1-19. DOI: 10.3390/toxins6010001

[161] Li Y, Wang Z, Beier RC, et al. T-2 toxin, a trichothecene mycotoxin: Review of toxicity, metabolism, and analytical methods. Journal of Agricultural and Food Chemistry. 2011; **59**:3441-3453

[162] Goswami RS, Kistler HC. Heading for disaster: *Fusarium graminearum* on cereal crops. Molecular Plant Pathology. 2004;**5**:515-525

[163] Palazzini JM, Ramirez ML, Torres AM, et al. Potential biocontrol agents for Fusarium head blight and deoxynivalenol production in wheat. Crop Protection. 2007;**26**:1702-1710

[164] Khan MR, Doohan FM. Bacterium-mediated control of Fusarium head blight disease of wheat and barley and associated mycotoxin contamination of grain. Biological Control. 2009;**48**:42-47

[165] Tian Y, Tan Y, Yan Z, et al. Antagonistic and detoxification potentials of Trichoderma isolates for control of Zearalenone (ZEN) producing *Fusarium graminearum*. Frontiers in Microbiology. 2018;**8**:2710

[166] Kosawang C, Karlsson M, Vélëz H, et al. Zearalenone detoxification by zearalenone hydrolase is important for the antagonistic ability of *Clonostachys rosea* against mycotoxigenic *Fusarium graminearum*. Fungal Biology. 2014;**118**:364-373

[167] Takahashi-Ando N, Kimura M, Kakeya H, et al. A novel lactonohydrolase responsible for the detoxification of zearalenone: Enzyme purification and gene cloning. The Biochemical Journal. 2002;**365**:1-6

[168] Takahashi-ando N, Ohsato S, Shibata T, et al. Metabolism of Zearalenone by genetically Modified organisms expressing the Detoxi cation gene from. Microbiology. 2004;**70**:3239-3245

[169] Karlsson M, Durling MB, Choi J, et al. Insights on the evolution of mycoparasitism from the genome of clonostachys rosea. Genome Biological Evolution. 2015;**7**:465-480

[170] Chatterjee S, Kuang Y, Splivallo R, et al. Interactions among filamentous fungi *Aspergillus niger*, *Fusarium verticillioides* and *Clonostachys rosea*: Fungal biomass, diversity of secreted metabolites and fumonisin production. BMC Microbiology. 2016;**16**:83

[171] Smith MC, Madec S, Coton E, et al. Natural co-occurrence of mycotoxins in foods and feeds and their in vitro combined toxicological effects. Toxins. 2016;**8**:94. DOI: 10.3390/toxins8040094

[172] Bayman P, Baker JL, Mahoney NE. Aspergillus on tree nuts: Incidence and associations. Mycopathologia. 2003;**155**:161-169

[173] Perrone G, Gallo A, Logrieco AF. Biodiversity of Aspergillus section Flavi in Europe in relation to the management of aflatoxin risk. Frontiers in Microbiology. 2014;**5**:377

[174] Niknejad F, Zaini F, Faramarzi M, et al. *Candida parapsilosis* as a potent biocontrol agent against growth and Aflatoxin production by *Aspergillus* species. Iran Journal of Public Health. 2012;**41**:72-80

[175] Jung B, Park SY, Lee YW, et al. Biological efficacy of *Streptomyces* sp. strain BN1 against the cereal head blight pathogen *Fusarium graminearum*. Plant Pathology Journal. 2013;**29**: 52-58

[176] Xue AG, Chen YH, Santanna SMR, et al. Efficacy of CLO-1 biofungicide in suppressing perithecial production by Gibberella zeae on crop residues. Canadian Journal of Plant Pathology. 2014;**36**:161-169

[177] Villaverde JJ, Sevilla-Morán B, Sandín-España P, et al. Biopesticides in the framework of the European pesticide regulation (EC) no. 1107/2009. Pest Management Science. 2014; **70**:2-5

[178] Brimner TA, Boland GJ. A review of the non-target effects of fungi used to biologically control plant diseases. Agriculture, Ecosystems and Environment. 2003;**100**:3-16

[179] Tijerino A, Hermosa R, Cardoza RE, Moraga J, Malmierca MG, Aleu J, Collado IG, Monte E, Gutierrez S. Overexpression of the *Trichoderma brevicompactum* tri5 gene: Effect on the expression of the trichodermin biosynthetic genes and on tomato seedlings. Toxins. 2011; **3**:1220-1232. DOI: 10.3390/toxins3091220

[180] Keswani C, Mishra S, Sarma BK, Singh SP, Singh HB. Unraveling the efficient applications of secondary metabolites of various *Trichoderma* spp. Applied Microbiology and Biotechnology. 2014;**98**:533-544. DOI: 10.1007/s00253-013-5344-5

[181] Berthiller F, Crews C, Dall'Asta C, Saeger SD, Haesaert G, Karlovsky P, Oswald IP, Seefelder W, Speijers G, Stroka J. Masked mycotoxins: A review. Molecular Nutrition & Food Research. 2013;**57**:165-186. DOI: 10.1002/mnfr.201100764

[182] Jestoi M. Emerging Fusarium -Mycotoxins Fusaproliferin, Beauvericin, Enniatins, and Moniliformin—A review. Critical Reviews in Food Science and Nutrition. 2008;**48**:21-49

[183] Abbas HK, Accinelli C, Thomas Shier W. Biological control of aflatoxin contamination in U.S. crops and the use of bioplastic formulations of *Aspergillus flavus* biocontrol strains to optimize application strategies. Journal of Agricultural and Food Chemistry. 2017;**65**: 7081-7087

[184] Mancini V, Romanazzi G. Seed treatments to control seedborne fungal pathogens of vegetable crops. Pest Management Science. 2014;**70**:860-868

[185] Audenaert K, Callewaert E, Höfte M, et al. Hydrogen peroxide induced by the fungicide prothioconazole triggers deoxynivalenol (DON) production by *Fusarium graminearum*. BMC Microbiology. 2010;**10**:112. DOI: 10.1186/1471-2180-10-112

[186] Mousa WK, Shearer C, Limay-Rios V, et al. Root-hair endophyte stacking in finger millet creates a physicochemical barrier to trap the fungal pathogen *Fusarium graminearum*. Nature Microbiology. DOI: 10.1038/nmicrobiol.2016.167

Chapter 5

Co-Occurrence of Mycotoxins and Its Detoxification Strategies

Mateen Abbas

Additional information is available at the end of the chapter

http://dx.doi.org/10.5772/intechopen.76562

Abstract

The contamination of foods and feeds by mycotoxins is significant problem worldwide that pose serious health hazardous effects in humans and animals. Risk arises from the fact that fungal species grow naturally in food and are difficult to eliminate. The presence of multiple mycotoxins (co-occurrence) in food products increases day by day and their natural co-occurrence is an increasing health concern due to the exposure of multiple fungal growth, which might exert greater toxicity than exposure of single mycotoxins. The presence of mycotoxins in food and feed are associated with health and reproductive issues, lower performance, and higher medical costs. Survey on co-occurrence of mycotoxins indicated that over 50% contaminated samples contained more than one mycotoxins and Asia faces a heightened risk of mycotoxins overall. There is a lack of information regarding co-occurrence of mycotoxins in food and animal feed. Face to this situation, the current chapter will be very informative to explore the incidence of multiple mycotoxins, their co-occurrence and the detoxification of mycotoxins using different techniques.

Keywords: mycotoxins, detoxification, food, feed, mitigation strategies

1. Introduction

Agricultural and Food commodities are highly susceptible to fungal growth in pre and post-harvest conditions as well as during storage. Different types of fungi especially belonging to the genus Aspergillus, Penicillium, Fusarium and Claviceps grow in crops, food and feed items throughout the world in favorable environmental conditions that ultimately produce a variety of toxins known as "Mycotoxins". The existence of more than one mycotoxin in food commodities is referred to as "Co-occurrence". Prominent mycotoxins occurring in agricultural commodities, include: aflatoxins (AFLA), ochratoxin A (OTA), zearalenone (ZEN), deoxynivalenol (DON), fumonisins (FUM) and T-toxin (T-2).

Foodstuffs are very prone to contaminants like bacteria and fungi in the pre-harvest and post-harvest stages especially, during storage when executed in poor conditions. These facts could be a cause of mycotoxins contamination in feeds and foods that pose serious health threat to animals and humans. Exposure of mycotoxins is a worldwide concern due to the globalization of food trade and its toxic nature. Some of these mycotoxins have hepatotoxic, nephrotoxic, immunosuppressive, genotoxic, teratogenic, and/or carcinogenic effects in human and animals. Consequently, mycotoxins have been a major concern of food regulatory authorities in all over the world about its exposure and hazardous nature in human and animals. Occurrence of multiple mycotoxins (co-occurrence) now gains much attention worldwide owing to its more toxic capacity (synergistic) as compared to single mycotoxin. According to the Biomin mycotoxins survey of 2015, more than 50% contaminated samples contained multiple mycotoxins in food and feed. Furthermore, co-occurrence of multiple mycotoxins increased from 2015 to 2016 and risk of mycotoxins is more heightened in Asia comparatively to other continents because of the favorable environmental conditions [1]. Frequency of mycotoxins produced by Fusarium fungal species comprising DON, FUM, ZEN are more frequent and co-occurrence of these mycotoxins can result severe detrimental impacts. The prevalence of mycotoxins in animal feed are associated with lower performance, poor growth, health and reproductive issues and higher medical costs for both animals and humans. Foods of animal origin are essential part of normal diet of everybody therefore; there is a need to assess co-occurrence of mycotoxins in animal feed and its counteracting strategies.

The worldwide contamination of agricultural commodities (crops, foods and feeds) with mycotoxins is a global concern that poses huge threat to animals and humans health. Contamination of foods by multiple mycotoxins not only has negative impact on health but also for global food security. Animal ingestion of contaminated feed with a variety of mycotoxins can result extensive damage to the liver, kidney and even induce cancer.

Mycotoxin contamination occurs widely in feedstuffs of plant origin, especially in cereals, seeds, fruits, fodder, agricultural feed or food intended for animal or human consumption [2–6]. Human beings are exposed by the effects of these toxins when used the foods of animal origin like milk, meat and eggs [7]. Furthermore, mycotoxins lead to massive economic losses, including loss of livestock production, loss of forage crops and feeds, and loss of human and animal life [8]. At the moment, different mycotoxins have been identified globally, and food regulatory authorities focused mainly on the potent and frequently present mycotoxins that have proven lethal. In continent Asia, ZEA, DON and FUM mycotoxins produced by fungal specie Fusarium are frequently present in animal feed elicit great health concerns to animals and humans due to their toxic effects [9, 10].

2. Co-occurrence of mycotoxins

Contamination of food commodities with fungus is commonly seen in every part of the world and it diverge from region to region depending upon the food products and environmental conditions like temperature & humidity. The diversity of fungi species grown on food products under various ecological conditions were observed that produce particular mycotoxins but it can occur singly or in multiple (co-occurrence). The co-occurrence of mycotoxins can affect both the production of mycotoxin and the toxicity of the contaminated material. Mycotoxins risk not only threatens the people living in tropical climate countries but it also be hazardous for people of temperate climates countries like United States of America and Europe.

During the last 10 years, incidence of multiple mycotoxins (AFLA, OTA, ZEN, DON and FUM) produced by different fungal species particularly Fusarium and Aspergillus genus have been reported in cereals from different countries [11–19]. Natural co-occurrence of mycotoxins in cereal-based infant products was also observed from Tunisia, where 32% samples were detected contaminated with multiple mycotoxins [20]. It was noticed that Fusarium fungal species can produce different mycotoxins simultaneously, and their co-occurrence became an important issue in the past years for risk assessment [21–23], these multiple toxins can have additive, antagonist or synergic effects [24, 25].

Global occurrence of mycotoxins in cereals and processed food products indicated that five major mycotoxins namely AFLA, OTA, ZEN, DON, FUM are mostly found during the past 10 years in these food stuffs. FUM mycotoxins were maximally detected (61%) in these cereals and processed foods, DON were identified in 58% samples and AFLA were noticed in 55% samples. However, contamination of ZEN and OTA in these food items were 46% and 29%, respectively [26]. It was also noticed that contamination of mycotoxins in processed food products were relatively less than the cereal grains. More than one mycotoxin can be produced by single of numerous fungal species and it may found in different combinations in food stuffs which may exert additive, antagonistic and synergistic effect in animals and humans.

Multiple occurrence (co-occurrence) of mycotoxins in European region revealed that AFLA and OTA mycotoxins were mostly found (24%) whereas the prevalence of other mycotoxins was comparatively less (Approx. 10%). Similarly, the co-occurrence of AFLA and OTA was highly detected (35%) in African countries and the occurrence of other combinations was comparatively fewer (29%). Conversely, in Asia FUM and AFLA combination was highly noticed (78%) and the prevalence of similar combination (FUM + AFLA) was found (50%) in South America, while FUM + ZEA was second most observed combination (25%) among other mycotoxins. In short, co-occurrence of AFLA and FUM mycotoxins was highly observed in Asia, Africa and South America [1, 15, 27–44].

Co-occurrence of different mycotoxins was noted in Solvak and observed the highest correlation between DON and Nivalenol toxins. On the other hand, no correlation between ZEA and DON was noticed [45].

According to the latest Biomin mycotoxin Survey (2016), DON and FUM are the most commonly found mycotoxins in feedstuffs, analyzed in 4027 animal feed samples and feed ingredients collected from >50 countries. The major food items collected in this survey include corn, wheat, barley, rice, soybean meal, corn gluten meal, dried distillers grains (DDGS) and silage, that are used in feed among others [46].

Out of all samples, DON were detected in 73%, FUM were found 64 and 53% samples were contaminated by ZEN. Whereas, contamination of AFLA were detected in 25%, T-2 toxins in 18 and 12% samples were found contaminated with OTA, shown in **Figure 1**.

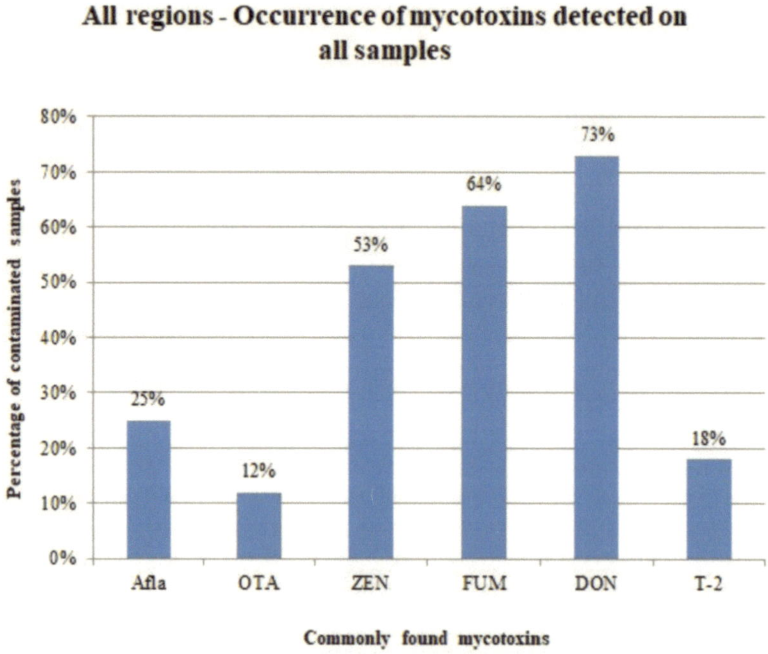

Figure 1. Worldwide occurrence of mycotoxins in food and feed surveyed in 2016.

According to the Biomin (An animal nutrition company) survey of 2017, 96% of all samples contaminated with at least one mycotoxins however, 75% samples contained two or more mycotoxins (**Figure 2**). However, survey of mycotoxins in poultry feed depicted that two-thirds (66%) poultry feed samples contained two or more mycotoxins and noted the highest mycotoxins risk (80%) in Asia comparatively to other continents [47].

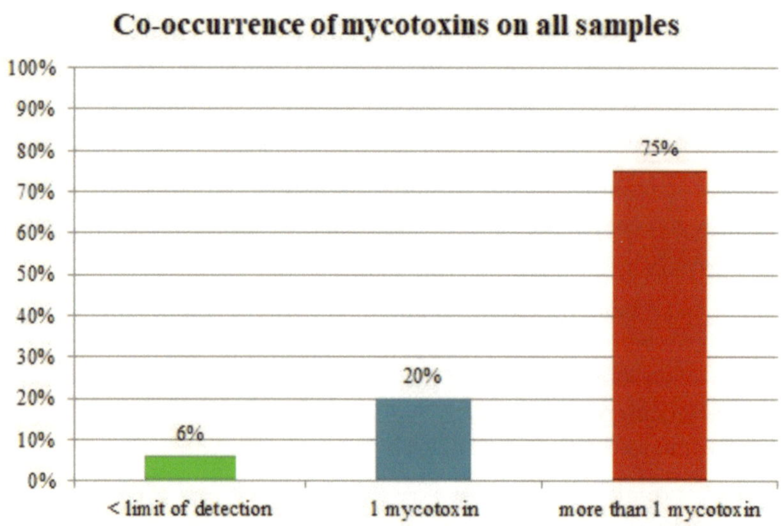

Figure 2. Co-occurrence of mycotoxins in food and feed commodities worldwide in 2017.

Worldwide contamination of mycotoxins in food commodities are represented in **Table 1** (BIOMIN World Mycotoxin survey, January to September, 2017).

It observed that, 84% of animal feed samples contaminated with single mycotoxins however more than 50% samples contaminated with several mycotoxins [1].

Multiple mycotoxin contamination may responsible of additional problems, like synergistic effects that exaggerate the more deleterious consequences for animals. The combination of DON and ZEN is reported synergistic pairing as stated by Dr. Timothy Jenkins who is product manager mycotoxins at animal nutrition company Biomin: "The effect of ZEN on reproductive systems can sometimes be worsened by the presence of DON."

2.1. Occurrence of mycotoxins in plant meals

2.1.1. Risk to aquaculture

The tendency and the economic need to replace the expensive fishmeal (an animal-derived proteins) with the cost-effective plant-based protein sources, has increased the impact of mycotoxins contamination in aquaculture feeds [48]. Mycotoxins have negative impact not only on the performance and health of terrestrial livestock species but it can also be lethal for aquaculture species [49, 50]. Mycotoxins effects even become more important in aquaculture sector due to the escalating cost of fishmeal and the necessity to pinpoint and use more cost-effective protein sources such as plant protein or other plant based products. Toxic fungal metabolites that probably affect the aquaculture species are produced mainly by Fusarium, Aspergillus and Penicillium species. Toxins produce by these fungal species are known to be carcinogenic (e.g., AFLA, OTA, FUM), hepatotoxic (e.g., AFLA), nephrotoxic (e.g., OTA), estrogenic (e.g., ZEN), dermatotoxic (e.g., trichothecenes) and immunosuppressive (e.g., AFLA, OTA and T-2 toxin).

According to the latest Biomin survey of 2107, it was found that Fusarium mycotoxins were the most prevalent mycotoxin worldwide among the other mycotoxins (AFLA, OTA, ZEN, DON, FUM and T-2 toxins) followed by AFLA. Analysis were performed in 8345 plant meal samples including corn, corn DDGS, corn gluten meal, wheat, wheat bran, rice, rice bran and soybean meal for detection of mycotoxins collected from different regions all over the world [47, 51, 52]. Corn gluten meal and corn DDGS which are commonly used in aquaculture feed were found highly contaminated with DON and FUM.

Some marine species (especially rainbow trout and *Litopenaeus vannamei*) are known to be sensitive for FUM that may cause variation in sphingolipid metabolism and inducing cancer [53–55]. FUM obstruct the sphinganine (sphingosine) N-acyl transferase (ceramide synthase), a key enzyme in lipid metabolism, resulting in the disruption of this pathway. DON, was particularly found most prevalent mycotoxins in rainbow trout (*Oncorhynchus mykiss*) responsible for decreases in growth, feed intake, feed efficiency and energy utilization [56].

Co-occurrence of mycotoxin was also noted in plant meals commonly used in aquaculture potentially leading to synergistic or additive effects. Approximately, 74% samples were contaminated with two or more mycotoxins as depicted by latest Biomin survey (2017) that can lead to significant economic impacts in the aquaculture sector [47].

Continents	Occurrence of Mycotoxins											
	AFLA		ZEN		DON		T-2		FUM		OTA	
	% contaminated samples	Average of positives (ppb)	% contaminated samples	Average of positives (ppb)	% contaminated samples	Average of positives (ppb)	% contaminated samples	Average of positives (ppb)	% contaminated samples	Average of positives (ppb)	% contaminated samples	Average of positives (ppb)
South and Central America	25	8	49	118	84	898	26	39	77	3227	4	3
North America	4	19	51	226	78	1112	3	41	60	1829	7	5
Europe	18	4	52	54	72	448	35	37	50	582	27	9
Asia	34	63	48	202	78	788	3	55	82	1026	27	8
Middle East	13	4	53	134	69	719	11	25	68	873	30	2
Africa	12	19	38	130	71	510	1	26	66	1221	14	4

Table 1. Worldwide contamination of mycotoxins in food commodities (2017).

2.2. Mycotoxin's effect in poultry

Prevalence of coccidiosis is common disease in broilers responsible for big loss (US$5–6 billion) globally each year. Coccidiosis is a renowned influencing factor for necrotic enteritis and predicted to cost poultry sector US$3 billion per annum. Existence of mycotoxins in poultry feeds aggravates coccidiosis in poultry; even its small amount can increase Eimeria infection and disease sternness in Poultry. Stakeholders in poultry sector always looking to minimize the effect of coccidiosis on their flocks.

Factors responsible for mycotoxins' intensification of coccidiosis include mycotoxin contamination in feed, higher immunosuppressive effects on broilers, and the possible synergistic effects between mycotoxins.

Aftereffects of FUM and DON toxins can be worse even if present in small concentration allowed by US and European guidelines. Permissible levels set by US FDA for FUM and DON are 30 and 10 ppm for poultry feed, respectively. However, allowed limits adapted by European regulations for FUM (20 ppm) and DON (5 ppm) toxins in poultry feeds are somewhat more stringent relatively to American regulations. FUM and DON may have some synergistic effects known to inhibit some vital functions of cells, interrupt intestinal cells that work as a barrier between pathogen and bodies of bird [57].

2.3. Impact of mycotoxins in livestock

Mycotoxins residues in food of animal origin like milk, meat (tissues) and eggs are frequently reported in every region. AFLA not only evidenced as hepato-toxic but it also have some other toxic effects like carcinogenic, mutagenic and teratogenic properties for humans as well as animals. Evidence of AFLA residues has been found so far in milk, meat tissue and eggs. Most importantly AFLA residues frequently found in milk as AFLA M1 and M2, which are the metabolites of AFLA B1 and B2. These toxic metabolites are produced when dairy animals fed on AFLA contaminated feed. It was noticed that concentrated animal feed (e.g., cotton seed cake, maize oil cake) was mostly found contaminated with huge level of mycotoxins. Conversion of AFLA B1 and B2 into the AFLA M1 and M2 in dairy animals are linearly dependent on the intake of contaminated feed and the toxin elimination totally from animal body usually finished 3 days after withdrawal of contaminated feed. The ratio between ingested and excreted AFLA is usually 1–3%, but it can be 6% presuming worst case scenarios [58–60]. Carry-over (or residues) of mycotoxins especially AFLA in milk is highly focused as it's routinely used by everyone in every part of the world especially children's and infants [61].

According to the latest mycotoxin survey it was noted that the risk levels are certainly elevated in many regions of the world. Globally, the average risk level was 62%, ranged from 46% (in Middle East) to 80% (in Asia). In light of the latest mycotoxin results, Dr. Timothy Jenkins, Mycotoxin Risk Management Product Manager at Biomin states that "livestock producers and stakeholders should be vigilant in monitoring their feed and feed ingredients for mycotoxins," [62].

Approximately, two-thirds contaminated samples contained more than one mycotoxins in animal feed and it observed that particular type of mycotoxins and its concentration vary due to climate, weather patterns and seasonal shifts, etc."

2.4. Climate change and its impact on mycotoxins

Temperature and humidity are two main factors that boost up the fungal growth and production of mycotoxins. As the world climate fluctuating, the pattern of mycotoxins contamination also vicissitudes, accordingly. The Intergovernmental Panel on Climate Change (IPCC) reported (2014) the different global warming projections and predict that global temperatures may increase by up to 4.8°C in the year 2100. Climate change will definitely affect the agriculture sector, variations in temperature and humidity may affect the efficacy of pesticide and fungicide applications, life-cycle of insects that promote fungal infections of crops may alter as well. On the other hand, fungal species may displace by other more aggressive or virulent fungi due to change in climate. If temperature begins to rise in upcoming years then the highest mycotoxin risks will be observed not only in countries with tropical climates but also in countries with temperate climates, such as parts of Europe and the United States of America [63–65].

3. Counteracting strategies

Dr. Timothy Jenkins stated that "Avoidance of contaminated food & feed and attention to storage conditions are logical approaches to reducing the mycotoxin risk."

Prevention and detection is the reliable approach with regular application of mycotoxin absorbents to minimize its lethal effects [62].

3.1. Decontamination or detoxification of mycotoxins

To minimize the level of mycotoxins in food and feed, several efforts have been made both In-vitro (in raw material and processed food) and In-vivo (within animal body). Generally, mycotoxin removal strategies can be divided in two phases, pre-harvest treatment to control or inhibit the growth of fungus and post-harvest remediation of contaminated commodities. However, preventive approaches such as plant disease management, good agricultural practices and adequate storage conditions might control the mycotoxin levels in food commodities but are not always sufficient to eradicate mycotoxins completely. Therefore, economically suitable and practically applicable approaches are required to decontaminate or detoxify the mycotoxins in food chain [66–68].

Ideally, the detoxification strategy should have the following properties: (1) inactivate, destroy or remove mycotoxin, (2) non-toxic, (3) easy or handy, (4) economical, (5) retain the nutritive value. In addition to these properties, the process should be field oriented and inexpensive.

Degradation or detoxification of toxic fungal metabolites may be an ideal approach to remove or decontaminate the toxins form food and feed products if the process not alters its nutritional composition. As most mycotoxins exhibit a high chemical stability, development of degradation or decontamination methods compatible with food quality standards is a challenging task and researchers still working to optimize the more efficient and appropriate process. Over the last decades biological, chemical and physical strategies for the degradation and decontamination of mycotoxins were investigated extensively [67, 69, 70]. Physical tactics mainly include washing, heating and irradiation were studied. Different mycotoxin binders (organic and mineral) were tried for the removal of toxic metabolites and considered the more effective removal process of mycotoxins from foodstuffs. More recently biological, enzymatic and chemical degradation procedures were also investigated and found effective. Chemical degradation processes comprise, application of acids, bases, chlorinating agents, oxidizing agents, formaldehyde and ammoniation were studied in food commodities [67, 70].

3.2. Physical methods of degradation

Removal of mycotoxins by physical approaches comprised sorting, dehulling, cleaning, milling, heating and irradiation or combinatorial methods. Organic, inorganic or mineral binders are also being tried for the decontamination of mycotoxins, although these adsorbing binders have some promising features, some may have adverse nutritional effects due to binding capacity of minerals and vitamins [71–82].

Technical plasma is a latest and innovative physical approach for the removal of mycotoxins from food and feed. Latest application of cold atmospheric pressure plasma (CAPP) in demolition of plant pathogens indicated that the process is appropriate for sensitive biological stuffs. Different types of plasma were used effectively for inhibition of fungal growth and for the decontamination of mycotoxins [83–88]. Recently, studies indicated that CAPP capable to degrade the mycotoxins in cereals and grains very efficiently [89].

3.3. Chemical methods of degradation

Degradation of mycotoxins can also be attained via chemical reactions. Different chemicals processes like hydrolysis, ammoniation, ozonation, peroxidation, and the use of hydrochloric acid, ascorbic acid, sodium bisulfite, hydrogen peroxide, formaldehyde, ammonia, ammonium hydroxide and are reported in different studies to decontaminate the mycotoxins in food [90]. However, chemical degradation does not fulfill the recommended criteria of FAO because some chemicals produce toxic metabolites and reduce the nutritional values of foodstuffs [91–93].

3.4. Biological degradation

Physical and chemical degradation methods have some confines such as losses in the nutritional value, limited efficacy and safety issues, in addition of these shortcomings costly equipment required to accomplish these techniques. Biological degradations are considered superb as it works under environment friendly conditions. Microbial degradations of mycotoxins are also preferred, since it can be a specific, efficient, environment friendly, irreversible and non-toxic. Degradation of mycotoxins using fungi are not considered a best choice because of its complicated procedures and long incubation time. However, bacterial degradation of mycotoxins has promising applications due to the high degradation rate and wide reaction conditions. Detoxification process using probiotic bacteria is also trying, which can be directly applied in the foodstuffs. Furthermore, the use of enzymes appears to be an auspicious choice for detoxification of mycotoxins [94, 95].

4. Conclusions

The current chapter contributes to increase the knowledge concerning the co-occurrence of mycotoxins in food commodities. It was noticed that co-occurrence of mycotoxins were exist in food and feed items of almost every country however, the occurrence vary from region to region. Prevalence and frequency of the mycotoxins are correlated with the locality and weather parameters (rainfall, humidity and temperatures). It would be more important that legislation of respective countries should be more stringent to protect the consumers from the lethal effects of mycotoxins.

Acknowledgements

I would like to thank the Director, Quality Operations Laboratory (QOL), University of Veterinary and Animal Sciences (UVAS) and all colleagues for helpful suggestions and support in the preparation of manuscript.

Conflict of interest

The author declares that there is no conflict of interest.

Author details

Mateen Abbas

Address all correspondence to: mateen.abbas@uvas.edu.pk

Quality Operations Laboratory (QOL), University of Veterinary and Animal Sciences (UVAS), Lahore, Pakistan

References

[1] BIOMIN. Science & Solutions. Herzogenburg, Austria: BIOMIN Holding GmbH; 2015

[2] Guan S, Yin Y, Zhou T, Xie M, Ruan Z, Young JC. Microbial strategies to control aflatoxins in food and feed. World Mycotoxin Journal. 2011;**4**:413-424

[3] Wu L, Wang W, Yao K, et al. Effects of dietary arginine and glutamine on alleviating the impairment induced by deoxynivalenol stress and immune relevant cytokines in growing pigs. PLoS One. 2013;**8**:e69502

[4] Wu M, Xiao H, Ren W, Yin J, HuJiayu DJ, et al. An NMR-based metabolomic approach to investigate the effects of supplementation with glutamic acid in piglets challenged with deoxynivalenol. PLoS One. 2014;**9**:0113687

[5] Wu L, Liao P, He LQ, et al. Growth performance, serum biochemical profile, jejunal morphology, and the expression of nutrients transporter genes in deoxynivalenol (DON)-challenged growing pigs. BMC Veterinary Research. 2015a;**11**:144-154

[6] Li LP, He L, Feng Z, Ren W, Yin J, et al. Dietary LArginine supplementation protects weanling pigs from deoxynivalenol-induced toxicity. Toxins. 2015;**7**:1341-1354

[7] Council for Agricultural Science and Technology (CAST). Mycotoxins: Risks in Plant, Animal, and Human Systems. Ames, IA: Council for Agricultural Science and Technology; 2002

[8] Mohamed EZ. Impact of mycotoxins on humans and animals. Journal of Saudi Chemical Society. 2011;**15**(2):129-144

[9] Oueslati S, Romero-Gonzalez R, Lasram S, Frenich AG, Vidal JLM. Multi-mycotoxin determination in cereals and derived products marketed in Tunisia using ultrahigh performance liquid chromatography coupled to triple quadrupole mass spectrometry. Food and Chemical Toxicology. 2012;**50**(7):2376-2381

[10] Miazzo R, Dalcero A, Rosa CA, De Queiroz Carvalho EC, Magnoli C, Chiacchiera SM, et al. Efficacy of synthetic zeolite to reduce the toxicity of aflatoxin in broiler chicks. Poultry Science. 2000;**79**(1):1-6

[11] Ibanez-Vea M, Corcuera LA, Remiro R, Murillo-Arbizu MT, González-Penas E, Lizarraga E. Validation of a UHPLC-FLD method for the simultaneous quantification of aflatoxins, ochratoxin A and zearalenone in barley. Food Chemistry. 2011a;**127**(1):351-358

[12] Ibanez-Vea M, Martinez R, Gonzalez-Penas E, Lizarraga E, Lopez de Cerain A. Co-occurrence of aflatoxins, ochratoxin A and zearalenone in breakfast cereals from spanish market. Food Control. 2011b;**22**(12):1949-1955

[13] Montes R, Segarra R, Castillo MA. Trichothecenes in breakfast cereals from the Spanish retail market. Journal of Food Composition and Analysis. 2012;**27**:38-44

[14] Iqbal SZ, Rabbani T, Asi MR, Jinap S. Assessment of aflatoxins, ochratoxin A and zearalenone in breakfast cereals. Food Chemistry. 2014;**157**:257-262

[15] Villa P, Markaki P. Aflatoxin B1 and ochratoxin A in breakfast cereals from Athens market: Occurrence and risk assessment. Food Control. 2009;**20**(5):455-461

[16] Mahnine N, Meca G, Fernández-Franzón M, Manes J, Zinedine A. Occurrence of fumonisins B1, B2 and B3 in breakfast and infant cereals from Morocco. Phytopathologia Mediterranea. 2012;**51**(1):193-197

[17] Romagnoli B, Ferrari M, Bergamini C. Simultaneous determination of deoxynivalenol, zearalenone, T-2 and HT-2 toxins in breakfast cereals and baby food by high-performance liquid chromatography and tandem mass spectrometry. Journal of Mass Spectrometry. 2010;**45**(9):1075-1080

[18] Roscoe V, Lombaert GA, Huzel V, Neumann G, Melietio J, Kitchen D, Ellipsis Scott PM. Mycotoxins in breakfast cereals from the Canadian retail market: A 3-year survey. Food Additives & Contaminants: Part A. 2008;**25**(3):347-355

[19] Cunha SC, Fernandes JO. Development and validation of a method based on a QuEChERS procedure and heart-cutting GC-MS for determination of five mycotoxins in cereal products. Journal of Separation Science. 2010;**33**(4-5):600

[20] Oueslati S, Berrada H, Manes J, Juan C. Presence of mycotoxins in Tunisian infant foods samples and subsequent risk assessment. Food Control. 2018;**84**:362-369

[21] Alkadri D, Rubert J, Prodi A, Pisi A, Manes J, Soler C. Natural co-occurrence of mycotoxins in wheat grains from Italy and Syria. Food Chemistry. 2014;**157**:111-118

[22] Juan C, Covarelli L, Beccari G, Colasante V, Manes J. Simultaneous analysis of twenty-six mycotoxins in durum wheat grain from Italy. Food Control. 2016;**62**:322-329

[23] Juan C, Ritieni A, Manes J. Occurrence of Fusarium mycotoxins in Italian cereal and cereal products from organic farming. Food Chemistry. 2013;**141**(3):1747-1755

[24] Prosperini A, Font G, Ruiz MJ. Interaction effects of Fusarium enniatins (A, A1, B and B1) combinations on in vitro cytotoxicity of Caco-2 cells. Toxicology In Vitro. 2014;**28**(1):88-94

[25] Ruiz MJ, Macakova P, Juan-Garcia A, Font G. Cytotoxic effects of mycotoxin combinations in mammalian kidney cells. Food and Chemial Toxicology. 2011;**49**(10):2718-2724

[26] Lee HJ, Dojin R. Worldwide occurrence of mycotoxins in cereals and cereal-derived food products: Public health perspectives of their co-occurrence. Journal of Agricultural and Food Chemistry. 2017;**65**(33):7034-7051

[27] Sultana N, Rashid A, Tahira I, Hanif HU, Hanif NQ. Distribution of various mycotoxins in compoundvfeed, total mix ration and silage. Pakistan Veterinary Journal. 2013

[28] Sun G, Wang S, Hu X, Su J, Zhang Y, Xie Y, Zhang H, Tang L, Wang JS. Co-contamination of aflatoxin B1 and fumonisin B1 in food and human dietary exposure in three areas of China. Food Additives & Contaminants. Part A, Chemistry, Analysis, Control, Exposure & Risk Assessment. 2011;**28**:461-470

[29] Tanaka T, Yamamoto S, Hasegawa A, Aoki N, Besling JR, Sugiura Y, Ueno Y. A survey of the natural occurrence of Fusarium mycotoxins, deoxynivalenol, nivalenol and zearalenone, in cereals harvested in the Netherlands. Mycopathologia. 1990;**110**:19-22

[30] Tanaka T, Hasegawa A, Yamamoto S, Sugiura Y, Ueno Y. A case report on a minor contamination of nivalenol in cereals harvested in Canada. Mycopathologia. 1988;**101**:157-160

[31] Ueno Y, Iijima K, Wang SD, Sugiura Y, Sekijima M, Tanaka T, Chen C, Yu SZ. Fumonisins as a possible contributory risk factor for primary liver cancer: A 3-year study of corn harvested in Haimen, China, by HPLC and ELISA. Food and Chemical Toxicology. 1997;**35**:1143-1150

[32] Varga E, Glauner T, Berthiller F, Krska R, Schuhmacher R, Sulyok M. Development and validation of a (semi-)quantitative UHPLC-MS/MS method for the determination of 191 mycotoxins and other fungal metabolites in almonds, hazelnuts, peanuts and pistachios. Analytical and Bioanalytical Chemistry. 2013;**405**:5087-5104

[33] Vargas EA, Preis RA, Castro L, Silva CM. Co-occurrence of aflatoxins B1, B2, G1, G2, zearalenone and fumonisin B1 in Brazilian corn. Food Additives and Contaminants. 2001;**18**:981-986

[34] Vrabcheva T, Usleber E, Dietrich R, Martlbauer E. Co-occurrence of ochratoxin A and citrinin in cereals from Bulgarian villages with a history of Balkan endemic nephropathy. Journal of Agricultural and Food Chemistry. 2000;**48**:2483-2488

[35] Wang DS, Liang YX, Chau NT, Dien LD, Tanaka T, Ueno Y. Natural co-occurrence of Fusarium toxins and aflatoxin B1 in com for feed in North Vietnam. Natural Toxins. 1995;**3**:445-449

[36] Yamashita A, Yoshizawa T, Aiura Y, Sanchez PC, Dizon EI, Arim RH, Sardjono. Fusarium mycotoxins (fumonisins, nivalenol, and zearalenone) and aflatoxins in corn from Southeast Asia. Bioscience, Biotechnology, and Biochemistry. 1995;**59**:1804-1807

[37] Yoshizawa T, Yamashita A, Chokethaworn N. Occurrence of fumonisins and aflatoxins in corn from Thailand. Food Additives and Contaminants. 1996;**13**:163-168

[38] Zinedine A, Brera C, Elakhdari S, Catano C, Debegnach F, Angelini S, De Santis B, Faid M, Benlemlih M, Minardi V, Miraglia M. Natural occurrence of mycotoxins in cereals and spices commercialized in Morocco. Food Control. 2006;**17**:868-874

[39] Merhej J, Richard-Forget F, Barreau C. Regulation of trichothecene biosynthesis in Fusarium: Recent advances and new insights. Applied Microbiology and Biotechnology. 2011;**91**:519-528

[40] Gareis M, Zimmerman C, Schothorst R, Paulsch W, Vidnes A, Bergsten C, Paulsen B, Brera C, Maraglia M, Grossi S, et al. Collection of Occurrence Data of Fusarium Toxins in Food and Assessment of Dietary Intake by the Population of EU Member States; Directorate-General Health and Consumer Protection: Kulmbach, Germany; Berlin, Germany; Bilthoven, The Netherlands; Oslo, Norway; Rome, Italy; 2003. 606 p

[41] Miraglia M, Brera C. Assessment of Dietary Intake of Ochratoxin A by the Population of EU Member States; Directorate-General Health and Consumer Protection: Rome, Italy; 2002. 153 p

[42] Bennett JW, Klich M. Mycotoxins. Clinical Microbiology Reviews. 2003;**16**:497-516

[43] Pereira VL, Fernandes JO, Cunha SC. Mycotoxins in cereals and related foodstuffs: A review on occurrence and recent methods of analysis. Trends in Food Science and Technology. 2014;**36**:96-136

[44] Paterson RRM, Lima N. How will climate change affect mycotoxins in food? Food Research International. 2010;**43**:1902-1914

[45] Lacko-Bartoeova M, Jaroslav R, Lucia L. Fusarium mycotoxin contamination and co-occurrence in Slovak winter wheat grains. Zemdirbyste-Agriculture. 2017;**104**(2):173-178

[46] BIOMIN. Science & Solutions. Herzogenburg, Austria: BIOMIN Holding GmbH; 2016

[47] BIOMIN. Science & Solutions. Herzogenburg, Austria: BIOMIN Holding GmbH; 2017

[48] Gonçalves RA, Schatzmayr D, Hofstetter U, Santos GA. Occurrence of mycotoxins in aquaculture: Preliminary overview of Asian and European plant ingredients and finished feeds. World Mycotoxin Journal (In Press); 2017. p. 1-12

[49] D'Mello JPF, Macdonald AMC. Mycotoxins. Animal Feed Science and Technology. 1997;**69**:155-166

[50] Rotter BA, Prelusky DB, Pestka JJ. Toxicology of deoxynivalenol (vomitoxin). Journal of Toxicology and Environmental Health. Part A. 1995;**48**:1-34

[51] Richard J. Sampling and sample preparation for mycotoxin analysis. In: Romer Labs Guide to Mycotoxins. Romer Lab Union. 2000

[52] Binder EM, Tan LM, Chin LJ, Handl J, Richard J. Worldwide occurrence of mycotoxins in commodities, feeds and feed ingredients. Animal Feed Science and Technology. 2007;**137**:265-282

[53] Meredith FI, Riley RT, Bacon CW, Williams DE, Carlson DB. Extraction, quantification, and biological availability of fumonisin B1 incorporated into the Oregan test diet and fed to rainbow trout. Journal of Food Protection. 1998;**61**:1034-1038

[54] Riley RT, Enongene E, Voss KA, Norred WP, Meredith FI, Sharma RP, Spitsbergen J, Williams DE, Carlson DB, Merrill-Jr AH. Sphingolipid perturbations as mechanisms for fumonisin carcinogenesis. Environmental Health Perspectives. 2001;**109**:301-308

[55] Garcia-Morales MH, Perez-Velazquez M, Gonzalez-Felix ML, Burgos-Hernandez A, MO C-R, Bringas-Alvarado L, Ezquerra-Brauer JM. Effects of fumonisin B1-containing feed on the muscle proteins and ice-storage life of white shrimp (*Litopenaeus vannamei*). Journal of Aquatic Food Product Technology. 2103;**24**:340-353

[56] Hooft JM, Elmor A, Ibraheem EH, Encarnacao P, Bureau DP. Rainbow trout (*Oncorhynchus mykiss*) is extremely sensitive to the feed-borne Fusarium mycotoxin deoxynivalenol (DON). Aquaculture. 2011;**311**:224-232

[57] Starkl V. The Latest in Mycotoxin Risk Management in Poultry. MSc—Product Manager, Mycotoxin Risk Management. Science & Solutions No. 47—Poultry. 2017. (www.biomin.net)

[58] Ruangwises S, Ruangwises N. Occurrence of Afla-toxin M1 in pasteurized milk of the school milk project in Thailand. Journal of Food Protection. 2009;**72**(8):1761-1763

[59] Battacone G, Nudda A, Cannas A, Borlino AC, Bomboi G, Pulina G. Excretion of Aflatoxin M1 in milk of dairy ewes treated with different doses of Aflatoxin B1. Journal of Dairy Science. 2003;**86**(8):2667-2675. DOI: 0.3168/jds.S0022-0302(03)73862-4

[60] Opinion of the Scientific Panel on Contaminants in Food Chain on a Request From the Commission Related to Aflatoxin B1 as Undesirable Substance in Animal Feed. Request No. EFSA-Q-2003-035, The EFSA Journal. 2004;**39**:1-27

[61] Meucci V, Razzuoli E, Soldani G, Massart F. Mycotoxin detection in infant formula milks in Italy. Food Additives and Contaminant. Part A, Chemistry, Analysis, Control, Exposure & Risk Assessment. 2010;**27**(1):64-71

[62] Jenkins T, Mycotoxin survey: Co-occurrence still an issue. Product Manager, Mycotoxins. Erber Campus 1, 3131 Getzersdorf, Austria: Biomin Holding GmbH; 2017

[63] Kovalsky P. Climate change and mycotoxin prevalence. Broadening Horizons N°8, Product Manager Mycofix®, BIOMIN Holding GmbH. May 2014:6

[64] Rodrigues I, Naehrer K. A three-year survey on the worldwide occurrence of mycotoxins in feedstuffs and feed. Toxins. 2012;**4**:663-675. DOI: 10.3390/toxins4090663

[65] Streit E, Schwab C, Sulyok M, Naehrer K, Krska R, Schatzmayr G. Multi-Mycotoxin screening reveals the occurrence of 139 different secondary metabolites in feed and feed ingredients. Toxins. 2013;**5**(3):504-523. DOI: 10.3390/toxins5030504

[66] Zhu Y, Hassan Y, Watts C, Zhou T. Innovative technologies for the mitigation of mycotoxins in animal feed and ingredients a—Review of recent patents. Animal Feed Science and Technology. 2016;**216**:19-29

[67] Karlovsky P, Suman M, Berthiller F, De Meester J, Eisenbrand G, Perrin I, Oswald I, Speijers G, Chiodini A, Recker T, Dussort P. Impact of food processing and detoxification treatments on mycotoxin contamination. Mycotoxin Research. 2016;**32**:197-205

[68] Temba BA, Sultanbawa Y, Kriticos DJ, Fox GP, Harvey JJW, Fletcher MT. Tools for defusing a major global food and feed safety risk: Nonbiological postharvest procedures to decontaminate mycotoxins in foods and feeds. Journal of Agricultural and Food Chemistry. 2016;**64**:8959-8972

[69] He J, Zhou T, Young JC, Boland GJ, Scott PM. Chemical and biological transformations for detoxification of trichothecene mycotoxins in human and animal food chains: A review. Trends in Food Science and Technology. 2010;**21**:67-76

[70] Karlovsky P. Biological detoxification of fungal toxins and its use in plant breeding, feed and food production. Natural Toxins. 1999;**7**:1-23

[71] Scudamore KA, Baillie H, Patel S, Edwards SG. Occurrence and fate of Fusarium mycotoxins during commercial processing of oatsin the UK. Food Additives and Contaminants. 2007;**24**:1374-1385. DOI: 10.1080/02652030701509972

[72] Castells M, Ramos AJ, Sanchis V, Marín S. Distribution of total aflatoxins in milled fractions of hulled rice. Journal of Agricultural and Food Chemistry. 2007;**55**:2760-2764. DOI: 10.1021/jf063252d

[73] Khatibi PA, Berger G, Wilson J, Brooks WS, McMaster N, Griffey CA, et al. A comparison of two milling strategies to reduce the mycotoxin deoxynivalenol in barley. Journal of Agricultural and Food Chemistry. 2014;**62**:4204-4213. DOI: 10.1021/jf501208x

[74] Fandohan P, Ahouansou R, Houssou P, Hell K, Marasas WFO, Wingfield MJ. Impact of mechanical shelling and dehulling on Fusarium in fection and fumonisin contamination in maize. Food Additives and Contaminants. 2006;**23**:415-421. DOI: 10.1080/02652030500442516

[75] Rios G, Pinson-Gadais L, Abecassis J, Zakhia-Rozis N, Lullien-Pellerin V. Assessment of dehulling efficiency to reduced oxy nivalenol and Fusarium level in durum wheat grains. Journal of Cereal Science. 2009;**49**:387-392. DOI: 10.1016/j.jcs.2009.01.003

[76] Matumba L, VanPoucke C, Ediage EN, Jacobs B, DeSaeger S. Effectiveness of hand sorting, flotation/washing, dehulling and combinations thereof on the decontamination of mycotoxin-contaminated white maize. Food Additives & Contaminants. Part A, Chemistry, Analysis, Control, Exposure & Risk Assessment. 2015;**32**:960-969. DOI: 10.1080/19440049.2015.1029535

[77] Vander-Westhuizen L, Shephard GS, Rheeder JP, Burger HM, Gelderblom WCA, Wild CP, et al. Optimising sorting and washing of home-grown maize to reduce fumonisin contamination under laboratory-controlled conditions. Food Control. 2011;**22**:396-400. DOI: 10.1016/j.foodcont.2010.09.009

[78] Fandohan P, Zoumenou D, Hounhouigan DJ, Marasas WFO, Wingfield MJ, Hell K. Fate of aflatoxins and fumonisins during the processing of maize into food products in Benin. International Journal of Food Microbiology. 2005;**98**:249-259. DOI: 10.1016/j.ijfoodmicro.2004.07.007

[79] Ramos AJ, Finkgremmels J, Hernandez E. Prevention of toxic effects of mycotoxins by means of non-nutritive adsorbent compounds. Journal of Food Protection. 1996;**59**:631-641

[80] Kolosova A, Stroka J. Substances for reduction of the contamination of feed by mycotoxins: A review. World Mycotoxin Journal. 2011;**4**:225-256. DOI: 10.3920/WMJ2011.1288

[81] Huwig A, Freimund S, Kappeli O, Dutler H. Mycotoxin detoxication of animal feed by different adsorbents. Toxicology Letters. 2001;**122**:179-188. DOI: 10.1016/S0378-4274(01)00360-5

[82] Yiannikouris A, Bertin G, Jouany JP. Study of the adsorption capacity of Saccharomyces cerevisiae cell wall components toward mycotoxins and the chemical mechanisms invoked. Mycotoxin Factbook. 2006:347-361. DOI: 10.3920/978-90-8686-587-1

[83] Bormashenko E, Grynyov R, Bormashenko Y, Drori E. Cold radiofrequency plasma treatment modifies wettability and germination speed of plant seeds. Scientific Reports. 2012;**2**:741. DOI: 10.1038/srep00741

[84] Filatova I, Azharonok V, Kadyrov M, Belyavsky V, Gvodzdov A, Shik A, Antonuk A. The effect of plasma treatment of seeds of some grain and legumes on their sowing quality and productivity. Romanian Journal of Physics. 2011;**56**:139-143

[85] Avramidis G, Stuwe B, Richard W, Bellmann M, Stephan W, Von-Tiedemann A, Viol W. Fungicidal effects of an atmospheric pressure gas discharge and degradation mechanisms. Surface and Coating Technology. 2010;**205**:405-408

[86] Ouf SA, Basher AH, Mohamed AAH. Inhibitory effect of double atmospheric pressure argon cold plasma on spores and mycotoxin production of Aspergillus Niger contaminating date palm fruits. Journal of the Science of Food and Agriculture. 2015;**95**(15):3204-3210

[87] Park BJ, Takatori K, Sugita-Konishi Y, Kim IH, Lee MH, Han DW, Chung KH, Hyun SO, Park JC. Degradation of mycotoxins using microwave-induced argon plasma at atmospheric pressure. Surface and Coating Technology. 2007;**201**:5733-5737

[88] Zahoranova A, Henselova M, Hudecova D, Kalinakova B, Kovacik D, Medvecka V, Cernak M. Effect of cold atmospheric pressure plasma on the wheat seedlings vigor and on the inactivation of microorganisms on the seeds surface. Plasma Chemistry and Plasma Processing. 2015;**36**:397-414

[89] Bosch L, Katharina P, Georg A, Stephan W, Wolfgang V, Petr K. Plasma-based degradation of mycotoxins produced by Fusarium, Aspergillus and Alternaria species. Toxins. 2017;**97**(9):1-12

[90] Norred WP, Voss KA, Bacon CW, Riley RT. Effectiveness of ammonia treatment in detoxification of fumonisin contaminated corn. Food Chem.Toxicol. 1991;**29**:815-819. DOI: 10.1016/0278-6915(91)90108-J

[91] Hagler WM. Mycotoxins, cancer and health. In: Bray G, Ryan D, editors. Potential for Detoxification of Mycotoxin–Contaminated Commodities. Baton Rouge (La): Louisiana State University Press; 1991. pp. 253-269

[92] Young JC. Reduction in levels of deoxynivalenol on contaminated corn by chemical and physical treatment. Journal of Agricultural and Food Chemistry. 1986;**34**:465-467

[93] Young JC, Subryan LM, Potts D, McLaren ME, Gobran FH. Reduction in levels of deoxynivalenol in contaminated wheat by chemical and physical treatment. Journal of Agricultural and Food Chemistry. 1986;**34**:461-465

[94] Ji C, Yu F, Lihong Z. Review on biological degradation of mycotoxins. Animal Nutrition. 2016;**2**:127-133

[95] Schatzmayr G, Täubel M, Vekiru E, Moll D, Schatzmayr D, Binder EM, Krska R, Loibner AP. Detoxification of mycotoxins by biotransformation. In: Barug D, Bhatnagar D, Van Egmond HP, Vander-Kamp JW, Van- Osenbruggen WA, Visconti A, editors. The Mycotoxin Factbook, Food and Feed Topics. Wageningen, The Netherlands: Wageningen Academic Publishers; 2006. pp. 363-375

Chapter 6

Aflatoxin Management Strategies in Sub-Saharan Africa

Titilayo Falade

Additional information is available at the end of the chapter

http://dx.doi.org/10.5772/intechopen.78784

Abstract

Aflatoxins are natural poisons produced by some members of the *Aspergillus* section *Flavi* group. Their control is critical in sub-Saharan Africa as in other parts of the world because of the health and economic dangers that aflatoxins cause. Aflatoxin management requires a pipeline approach (from production to consumption) that addresses the pre-disposing factors to aflatoxin contamination. These strategies will involve strategies at the pre-harvest, peri-harvest and post-harvest stages to prevent contamination. Post-contamination practices are also relevant in situations where avoidance of contamination is not possible. Strategies that inform producers, handlers, consumers of what aflatoxins are, how they can be prevented from contaminating produce or managed are important for aflatoxin management. Additionally, the engagement public and private sectors, regional bodies and community associations are critical for effective aflatoxin management as they have the capacity to influence behavior changes and modulate practices that predispose food and feed to aflatoxin contamination. Furthermore, the role of research and academic institutions to provide factual information and effectively communicate technical information for aflatoxin management is crucial to avoid misinformation and application of improper practices.

Keywords: aflatoxin, management, Africa, *Aspergillus*, mycotoxins

1. Introduction

1.1. Aflatoxins and their impact on sub-Saharan Africa

Most parts of sub-Saharan Africa fall within the region of high perennial risk to mycotoxin contamination. This region is within 40°N and 40°S of the equator with warm and humid environmental conditions [1]. Under these favorable conditions of humidity and temperature, fungal prevalence is rife. Unfortunately, some fungi, as part of their metabolic processes, synthesize mycotoxins (fungal toxins), that contaminate crops intended for human and animal consumption [2]. Ingestion of contaminated crops results in morbidity and mortality where tolerable levels are exceeded in food and feed [3, 4]. Associated health dysfunctions caused by aflatoxin ingestion include liver carcinoma and other hepatic dysfunctions, stunting in children and associated cognitive deficiencies, reduced immunity, and ailments associated with nutrient malabsorption due to disruption to villi architecture [5–7]. Acute aflatoxin ingestion can result in death. In livestock, including poultry, swine and fishes, listlessness, poor feed conversion ratio, reduced productivity are additional signs of aflatoxin ingestion [8, 9].

In addition to the negative health impacts caused by aflatoxins, aflatoxins also limit income generation. This is because the import of aflatoxin-contaminated produce above regulatory limits of importing countries is prohibited. Therefore, aflatoxin contamination has been responsible for depriving the sub-Saharan region of trade opportunities. Also, trading relationships have been marred by notifications of consistent aflatoxin contamination such as through the rapid alert system of the European Union (https://ec.europa.eu/food/safety/rasff_en). Moreover, economies of households within the sub-Saharan region are negatively affected because household income is diverted in addressing morbidity caused by aflatoxicosis (illness caused by ingestion of aflatoxins) termed disability adjusted life years (DALYs) [10]. This reduces availability of income for more economically advantageous ventures. Therefore, aflatoxin management is critical for the health and economy of sub-Saharan Africa However, it is reported that countries build social networks of trading relationships based on achievable mycotoxin limits [11]. For example, France is a trading partner with the UK, Spain and Netherlands (among others) which have similar total aflatoxin standards of 4 ng/g. Similarly, the USA is a trading partner with Mexico, Colombia, Dominican Republic (and others) which have similar total aflatoxin standards of 20 ng/g in maize.

Aflatoxin management is critical also because in addition to environmental reasons for aflatoxin exposure, infrastructural deficits, informal market structures and improper cultural habits can introduce additional aflatoxin-exposure risks [12]. Management strategies therefore, of necessity requires multi-dimensional approaches that mitigate risks from multiple sources such as contamination risks during crop development, during harvesting and post-harvest. This chapter discusses the approaches that are necessary for aflatoxin mitigation, and those that have been used for the management of aflatoxins in sub-Saharan Africa and progress made so far. Brief mention is also made of emerging strategies for aflatoxin management.

1.2. Incidences of aflatoxicosis in sub-Saharan Africa

Aflatoxicosis may be broadly classified into **acute and chronic aflatoxicosis**. Acute aflatoxicosis refers to aflatoxin poisoning caused by ingestion of large doses of dietary aflatoxins. Chronic aflatoxicosis refers to aflatoxin poisoning caused by the ingestion of smaller amounts over extensive periods of time. Acute aflatoxicosis is severe often results in immediate fatalities. However, with chronic exposure the effects of exposure are cumulative, so exposure may be undetected in early stages because of its subsymptomatic nature. In sub-Saharan Africa, aflatoxin contamination has been reported by technical experts in academic journal and reports and by some news media outlets. Technical research has disclosed the prevalence and exposure levels in crops (e.g. maize, groundnuts, melon seeds (*egusi*), chillies, dried fish, local spices) [13–15]; in addition to biomarkers (e.g. those present in breastmilk of nursing mothers, blood serum and urine) [16, 17]. A comprehensive report of incidences have been reviewed [18]. These have revealed the presence of aflatoxins in food crops as an indicator of dietary exposure. These scientific studies have been conducted as part of academic programs, and developmental efforts in collaboration with national systems to establish exposure levels. They have majorly been for chronic exposures, and to provide empirical evidence for outbreaks caused by acute exposure. Incidences of chronic exposure are not as momentous as those for acute exposure, but they could be lifelong starting early in life. This is especially because exposure can precede birth, from foetal exposure through umbilical cord, to aflatoxin exposure very early in life (from the first 1000 days of life), via mothers' breastmilk (where the nursing mother has had dietary aflatoxin exposure), and through weaning foods made using contaminated food products [19]. Furthermore, in many parts of sub-Saharan Africa, staple food consumption is frequent and forms a constant source of dietary exposure to consumers. Limited diversity in the meals consumed increases exposure risk, especially if the food consumed is contaminated by these harmful toxins. Aside from the consumption of foods for dietary needs, recreational consumption of locally brewed beers is another risk factor contaminated cereals could form the stock material from which the brews are made from [20].

Converse to reports majorly on chronic exposure by technical experts, news media/communication expert reports are often based on acute exposure. Acute outbreaks have caused national alarm (such as those recorded in 1980, 2004 and 2012 in Kenya; and 2016 in Tanzania). These outbreaks of acute aflatoxicosis occurred due to the ingestion of unsuspectingly high levels of aflatoxins in maize consumed as a staple food Outbreaks were first reported as 'mysterious illness' or caused by 'toxic' or 'poisonous' food. This is due to the clandestine nature of aflatoxins. This bears similarity to the foremost global report of aflatoxicosis in 1960 called the "Turkey X' disease, where 'X' was the mysterious unknown [21]. The covert nature of aflatoxins is primarily because sensual perception of aflatoxins is nearly impossible since the toxins are invisible, tasteless and odorless when present in food crops. Management of aflatoxins during these times have called for crisis response actions that immediately forestall continued exposure.

2. Aflatoxin management strategies

Aflatoxin management requires multiple strategies including the following which are further discussed in details hereafter: Awareness of aflatoxins, Pre-harvest aflatoxin prevention/reduction, Peri-harvest aflatoxin prevention/reduction, Post-harvest aflatoxin prevention/reduction and Post-contamination aflatoxin management.

2.1. Awareness of aflatoxins

Awareness of aflatoxins is critical to its management because information is the basis for initiating and sustaining measures to control aflatoxin exposure and associated health and economic implications. Awareness is a result of access to available information. This knowledge helps to inform the general public, health care practitioners, social workers, policy makers and other stakeholders on the risks of mycotoxins and control strategies necessary for prevention of aflatoxicosis and post-contamination management of contaminated crops, where prevention of contamination is not possible. There are different schools of thought regarding the way awareness creation is most effective [22, 23]. One school of thought suggests that the focus should be a top-bottom approach in terms of awareness creation about the problems of and solutions to aflatoxins without a bottom-up approach. The argument for this is that all that is required by the general public is to understand that there are differences in food quality, rather than the technical details of aflatoxins. This system will require that a food grading system is in place that enables the lay buyer to make financial decisions based on product differentiation. Furthermore, this may be more effective in a more organized market system where product differentiation on price and quality attributes are easily discernable. Another school of thought suggests that awareness creation should be a combination of top-down and bottom-up approaches. The argument for this is that education of the lay person on the risks associated with aflatoxicosis is necessary for behavioral changes towards crop management practices. This is important given the informal systems of trading that occur at the rural levels. Furthermore, as the systems of crop management are varied and so may require specific changes in practices suited to the customs of the regions.

2.1.1. Multi-faceted aflatoxin-management strategies

Current efforts made on aflatoxin awareness have been via multiple channels including policy briefs, regional reports, traditional media and social media reports, and word-of-mouth by various bodies such as regional government bodies and government institutions, private-sector and commercial organizations, extension services and farmers groups/community societies, and academic and research institutions among others.

2.1.1.1. Regional governments and government institutions awareness

The most notable regional bodies in sub-Saharan Africa regarding aflatoxin management is the Partnership for Aflatoxin Control in Africa (PACA), established under the Africa Union at the 7th Comprehensive Africa Agriculture Development Program (CAADP). PACA has raised awareness at regional and national levels through programs such as Pan-African workshops (these workshops have brought together scientific experts, lay people, policy makers, farmers and industries), policy briefs, coordination of sensitization and surveillance exercises at regional and national levels (http://aflatoxinpartnership.org). Through PACA's efforts, which are often in partnership with key organizations involved in aflatoxin management/mitigation, policies requiring the control of aflatoxins in foods is becoming mainstream. In recent years (from 2014), PACA has implemented the Africa Aflatoxin Information Management System) (AfricaAIMS) in pilot countries (including Senegal, The Gambia, Malawi, Nigeria, Tanzania and Uganda) to collate and harmonize data on aflatoxins [24]. This has been useful for assisting countries to make definitive and coordinated efforts in aflatoxin surveillance and discussions for aflatoxin management.

http://dx.doi.org/10.5772/intechopen.78784

So far, technical reports form many of the reports on aflatoxins and aflatoxin management. There are concerns that these reports are too technical and so the dire messages of aflatoxin exposure, and beneficial information on relevant interventions for aflatoxin management may not reach all stakeholders. Infographics and short documentations via policy briefs such as those by PACA and the International Food Policy Research Institute (IFPRI) are being developed. These are deliberate measures that that have been taken for technical information to be readily grasped by lay readers/audiences and policy makers.

Other regionals communities involved with raising awareness on aflatoxin management in the sub-Saharan African region include Permanent Interstate Committee for Drought Control in the Sahel/Comité permanent inter-État de lutte contre la sécheresse au Sahel (CILSS), Common Market for Eastern and Southern Africa (COMESA) and Economic Community of West African States (ECOWAS). Regional governments and government institutions communities assist with the development of regulatory schemes and their enforcement, aflatoxin testing, development of infrastructure and trade relationships, coordinating the access to appropriate technologies and infrastructure and establishment of trade relationships. Awareness within the communities is also important for proper decision-making. This is done through workshops and meetings wherein technical experts can communicate the technical details in simpler terms and respond to queries to clear doubts.

2.1.1.2. Private-sector/commercial organizations

Private sector participation is key for aflatoxin management in the sub-Saharan Africa. This is particularly important because the private sector through demand-driven approach can influence the behaviors of growers, aggregators and important stakeholders towards adoption of aflatoxin management techniques. However, where there is no financial incentive or social incentive to change, growers' inertia to change can be high. The positive influence of the private sector in changing behaviors that promote aflatoxin accumulation have been demonstrated. A few examples are discussed here.

Example 1 – The World Food Program (WFP).

Through a scheme, Pay for Performance (P4P), the WFP provided food relief in danger and conflict prone-regions of the world and aided those economies in improving crop quality and reducing aflatoxin contamination [25]. P4P requires grains for food relief. Due to the need to procure high quality food materials for disaster relief and a desire to promote crop production and so aid the economies within such regions, WFP influenced growers' behaviors for reduced aflatoxin contamination. This improved grain quality in the market and introduced grading systems. Examples of countries where this project covered include Zambia, Tanzania, Ghana, Burkina Faso, Democratic Republic of Congo, Ethiopia. The project was implemented between 2008 and 2013 [25].

P4P operated via grassroot and growers' education on aflatoxin mitigation and measurement. Aflatoxin measurement in crops was done by using the blue box that contained aflatoxin test kits, moisture meter, sieves, in addition to other items. Due to the P4P scheme/initiative, WFP rejections of grains in market outlets decreased. WFP also paid a premium price above the prevailing market price to farmers who invested in behavior change as part of P4P. This percentage reduction demonstrated the power of influence that the private sector or those with high purchasing power can have on the market. A more detailed information on this program can be found at http://www1.wfp.org/purchase-for-progress. As part of the program under P4P, producers were trained on crop management practices at post-harvest such as rapid drying of grains to below 14% moisture content, grain sorting, proper sampling techniques for aflatoxin measurement, aflatoxin testing and sample grading. WFP purchased products from the farmers were possible and linked the farmers to markets for grains that they were unable to take up.

Example 2 – Nestlé Foods.

Mycotoxin screening, including screening for aflatoxins forms a critical component of Nestlé's quality assessment of raw materials. Like WFP, Nestlé has embarked on capacity development initiatives from farmers in out-grower schemes that they work with. This was the Grains Quality Improvement Project. Through training on crop management practices, including post-harvest management, Nestlé markedly reduced their rejection rate from 96 to 4% (between 2007 and 2017) in sub-Saharan countries such as Ghana where this concept has been applied [26]. The Grain Quality Improvement Project (2009) was conducted with the International Institute of Tropical Agriculture in Ghana, Nigeria and Côte D'Ivoire [27, 28]. This kind of initiative was imperative for an International Food Brand Nestlé. Additionally, it helped the company to continue to buy locally and at the desired quality. The social impact of this project was perhaps important for Nestle's cooperate social responsibility goals and for the brand to retain its competitive advantage while not reneging on the strict quality standards for its food grains.

Example 3 – AgResults Nigeria Aflasafe™ Pilot Program.

The private sector involvement via the AgResults Nigeria Aflasafe™ Pilot program was designed to incentivize the use of technologies and implement practices that reduce aflatoxin incidence in crop (http://agresults.org/en/283/). Aflasafe™ is a biological control technology that favors the proliferation of naturally occurring populations of non-aflatoxigenic *Aspergillus* strains through competitive exclusion of toxin-producing aflatoxigenic *Aspergilli* [29]. The AgResults Nigeria Aflasafe™ Pilot Program introduced in Nigeria in 2013 encourages private businesses, called (Aflasafe) Implementers, involved in coordinating farmers and aggregating farmers' produce to reduce aflatoxin prevalence in crops by providing the necessary skills and technical information for Implementers to do so via training workshops and linking them to markets seeking premium quality grains (via Innovation Platforms) [30]. The AgResults program operates in Nigeria and is specifically targeted at promoting the use of Aflasafe™ as an inclusion to the good agricultural practices provided in the training package.

The private sector's involvement via this pilot program is two-fold. (1) The farmers' grain purchase coordination through Implementers (private businesses that coordinate the training of aflatoxin management including the use of Aflasafe™) ensures that demand for high quality grains are accessible; and (2) Purchase of high quality grains by the food and feed industries (especially the poultry industry) drive the demand for high quality grains. These food and feed industries pay a premium price for the high-quality grains. Additionally, the implementers gain a premium for proper implementation of the aflatoxin-management practice [31]. Due to the sustained demand for high quality grain by the food and feed industries, the implementers maintain the demand for the use of Aflasafe as part of aflatoxin management practices. As such, with the modulation of *Aspergillus* populations through repeated use of Aflasafe demand for maize with safe levels of aflatoxins in maize grains where the market demands are met with a price incentive as a driver in a pull-mechanism for the implementation of aflatoxin management techniques and technologies.

2.1.1.3. Extension services and farmers groups/community societies

In many parts of sub-Saharan Africa, farmers rely on and trust extension officers as accurate and reliable sources of agricultural advice. Therefore, extension agents are a powerful source of knowledge dissemination and awareness creation. However, due to the limitations in budgetary allocations, extension officers do not always have the financial power to reach out to many farmers in the farming communities with up-to-date knowledge on skills and technologies. Additionally, budgetary constraint also limits the ability of the extension officers to regularly receive training required to update their knowledge, skills and practices.

Farming communities have started organizing themselves into community groups with leadership structures that help in information dissemination [32]. When training is received by leaders in these groups within a central location, they are then able to disseminate the information in their local chapters. Information about aflatoxin management in many occasions has reached farmers this way. Through these organizational structures, groups are also able to organize field days or famers field schools. Field days where demonstration plots are displayed to farmers also constitute a form of training regularly done. However, this is difficult for aflatoxin control demonstrations, since the chemical toxin is not perceptible with the senses.

2.1.1.4. Academic and research institutions

Academic and research institutions play a key role in creating awareness of the control strategies for aflatoxin and aflatoxicosis prevalence. It is important for them to share accurate information about the management of aflatoxins. Distorted or inaccurate information about aflatoxin management is detrimental to awareness creation efforts made towards aflatoxin mitigation. Academic and research institutions have contributed to raising awareness through the publication of technical reports, discussions at technical meetings and contributions to non-technical writings and reports. They also contribute by organizing training meetings for important stakeholder groups such as extension practitioners, farmers groups, the private sector, regulatory organizations, and other important stakeholders to attend. It is also important for educational institutions and research organizations to partner in training students on aflatoxin management and other phytopathology concerns. This may ensure continuity in capacity development for the management of aflatoxigenic fungi, their toxins and other food security and food safety threats.

2.1.1.5. Other awareness platforms

Online documentation (e.g. websites, blogs, social networks), field extension services, commercial organizations and word of mouth are also important avenues of awareness creation. Dissemination of information via traditional media such as newspaper publications, radio broadcasts and discussions are also important for ensuring that the population gets the required information and to gauge the level of awareness/responses to the sensitization efforts. It is important that these efforts continue where already in place and make-up concerted efforts that are contributory to awareness creation as an important aflatoxin management strategy.

2.2. Aflatoxin management

2.2.1. Pre-harvest aflatoxin prevention/reduction

Although pre-, peri, and post-harvest aflatoxin management strategies; have been itemized as different from awareness creation, knowledge of these strategies is important for awareness. For pre-harvest aflatoxin management to receive contextual appreciation it is important to understand how aflatoxin contamination occurs. Natural contamination of food by aflatoxins requires contamination by aflatoxigenic strains of *Aspergilli.* Aflatoxin-producing strains of the *Aspergillus* section *Flavi* group such as *Aspergillus flavus, A. parasiticus, A. nominus* and S strains are responsible for contamination. Recently, a novel aflatoxin producer called *A. korhogoensis* (defined as a "*a novel cryptic species within the A. flavus clade*" was identified in Côte d'Ivoire [33]. Route of contamination is typically one by which the spores of these strains can enter the grains. Fungal spores reside on crop debris, in soils and can be air-borne when dispersed by wind. Spores can also be carried by insects and birds directly to the grains and thereby contaminate them [34–36].

To this end, methods that serve as barriers in preventing aflatoxigenic fungi from gaining entrance into the crop are critical for the control of aflatoxin contamination. For the maize during crop development, spores can enter grains via the silk channel (each silk thread leads to a kernel of maize), through cracks in the kernel because of abiotic stress such as heat or drought, and biotic stresses such as insects or birds [34, 37]. Furthermore, reducing the populations of the aflatoxin-producers in the environment can also reduce the risk of human exposure to aflatoxin. Pre-harvest management of aflatoxin contamination therefore comprises:

- Breeding efforts that increase the barriers to aflatoxigenic fungi [38]. These have been explored through increased tightness of husk cover and increased hardness of grains. These reduce the possibility of fungal entry into the grain and therefore aflatoxin contamination. However, flint grains (very hard grains) are difficult to process and because of that, farmers are not always willing to grow these varieties. Gene silencing as a method for aflatoxin management was recently developed by the International Crops Research Institute for the Semi-Arid Tropics (ICRISAT) [39]. However, acceptance of genetic modification of foods in and for sub-Saharan Africa has not received wide acceptance.

- Insect and pest control reduces the populations of pests that pre-dispose the crop to aflatoxin contamination. Insect control is particularly very important because of the strong correlation between mycotoxin contamination and insect damage. Using pest control can significantly reduce the risk of associated mycotoxins. With the growing inclinations for organic farming globally, the use of non-synthetic pesticides is preferable. Bird scare to prevent damage to the crop is also important. These practices do not only address the risk of contamination but are also important for maintaining optimum yields.
- Biological control of aflatoxin is another pre-harvest control strategy that is being adopted in sub-Saharan Africa. Aflasafe as reviewed earlier is a biocontrol measure. It involves the use of non-toxin producing strains to compete with aflatoxin-producing strains on the field as a naturally occurring displacement strategy implemented about a fortnight before crop flowering. Native strains are isolated from regions where the product is to be applied to the most suited/adapted non-toxin producing strains to that environment through rigorous research efforts for isolate selection. The technology has been commercialized under the trade name Aflasafe in a few African countries with continuing research efforts [29].

While mold contamination is known in many parts of sub-Saharan Africa because of their visual presentation and bitter taste, the aflatoxins that they produce are frequently unknown because they lack sensory attributes. Therefore, moldy grains would attract lesser value, while grains without visible mold, are not necessarily without aflatoxin contamination. Therefore, it is not uncommon for these grains to be used in the processing of food or feed material in which mold appearance is masked. This is for instance, in the processing of peanut butter, groundnut cake, poultry feed and fermentation for beers [40–43]. However, this is not a good management technique for aflatoxins as these poor-quality grains enter the food chain as alternative food products and the processing techniques may either minimally reduce the aflatoxins or concentrate the aflatoxins. However, visual signs of mold are not the only indicators of fungal infestation. It is possible for strains that produce high levels of aflatoxins to mildly infected grains, resulting in high aflatoxin levels. Also, grains contaminated with aflatoxins that have been washed and dried after infection, may no longer have visible mold growth but still contain the aflatoxins. This is because aflatoxins are only very mildly soluble in water at 10 mg/ml and are heat stable up to 150°C, after which they are only mildly detoxified [44].

2.2.2. *Peri-harvest aflatoxin prevention/reduction*

During harvest, exposure to aflatoxin contamination can occur due to practices that expose the crop to aflatoxigenic fungi as it is harvested. These could include harvesting during the rains or during high moisture conditions that encourage fungal proliferation; harvesting into recycled or contaminated containers such as bags, and carts that harbor the toxigenic mold or insects, or directly onto uncovered ground surfaces, threshing during harvest in a way that damages the grains. Preventing these would therefore involve the use of clean surfaces or containers for placement of harvested grains and rapid drying after harvest to avoid incubation of the fungus and subsequent accumulation of the toxin.

2.2.3. *Post-harvest aflatoxin prevention/reduction*

Post-harvest practices occur immediately after harvesting grain produce. These practices are inclusive of practices undertaken such as transportation, storage and processing of the harvested agricultural produce. As with peri-harvest practices, it is important to prevent predisposing factors such as pest infestation, re-contamination from re-used bags or improperly sanitized vessels or vehicles. It is therefore critical to ensure proper pest control, good aeration by placing stored grains in dry and well aerated storehouses. The use of wooden pallets, and away from walls, rather than placing bags in direct contact with floor surfaces and walls limits aflatoxin accumulation in hot spots. Other important post-harvest practices for reducing contamination include winnowing and sorting of grains to remove low density materials and grains that tend to harbor high proportions of the contaminated material [45].

2.2.4. *Post-contamination aflatoxin management*

Post-contamination management strategies are implemented when all attempts of reducing aflatoxin levels to permissible limits have failed. It is not recommended as a strategy without attempts to prevent contamination. There are controversies surrounding the implementation of some of these practices for the management of aflatoxins. Some of the practices include dilution with non-contaminated grains to reduce bulk contamination, ammoniation [46], binding of aflatoxins using adsorbents or aflatoxin-binders used for animal feed [47], nixtamalization [48], grain fermentation, radiation (including solar radiation) [49], grading to allow higher levels for non-dairy ruminants up to permissible levels, or use as alternative non-food uses such as production of bio-ethanol.

2.3. Conclusion

Aflatoxin management, including continuous public awareness and monitoring is required both on-farm and off-farm. Awareness is a critical stage of management and covers pre-harvest, peri-harvest, post-harvest stages of crop production. Post-contamination options are the last alternative to aflatoxin management and is the least preferred method for aflatoxin management in food and feed grains due to other associated risks of contaminant fate. The most preferred method is to prevent entry of aflatoxin-producing fungal strains, then limiting the ability of contaminating aflatoxin-producing strains from synthesizing and accumulating the harmful toxins in food grains. With proper aflatoxin-management, health and income improvement will increase in sub-Saharan Africa – a region with a high perennial risk of aflatoxin exposure, thus boosting the health of the people within the region.

Conflict of interest

The author declares no conflict of interest. Replace the entirety of this text with the 'conflict of interest' declaration.

Author details

Titilayo Falade

Address all correspondence to: t.falade@cgiar.org

International Institute of Tropical Agriculture, Ibadan, Nigeria

References

[1] Strosnider H, Azziz-Baumgartner E, Banziger M, Bhat RV, Breiman R, Brune M-N, DeCock K, Dilley A, Groopman J, Hell K, Henry SH, Jeffers D, Jolly C, Jolly P, Kibata GN, Lewis L, Liu X, Luber G, McCoy L, Mensah P, Miraglia M, Misore A, Njapau H, Ong C-N, Onsongo MTK, Page SW, Park D, Patel M, Phillips T, Pineiro M, Pronczuk J, Rogers HS, Rubin C, Sabino M, Schaafsma A, Shephard G, Stroka J, Wild C, Williams JT, Wilson D. Public health strategies for reducing aflatoxin exposure in developing countries: A workgroup report. Environmental Health Perspectives. 2006;**114**:1898-1903. DOI: 10.1289/ehp.9302

[2] Coppock RW, Christian RRG, Jacobsen BJ. Aflatoxins. In Veterinary Toxicology: Basic and Clinical Principles; Gupta RC Ed. San Diego: Academic Press; 2012. pp. 1181-1199. DOI: 10.1016/b978-0-12-385926-6.00102-2

[3] CDC Outbreak of Aflatoxin Poisoning–Eastern and Central Provinces, Kenya, Morb. Mortal. Wkly. Rep. January to July 2004;**53**:790-793

[4] Liu Y, Wu F. Global burden of aflatoxin-induced hepatocellular carcinoma: A risk assessment. Environmental Health Perspectives. 2010;**118**:818-824. DOI: 10.1289/ehp.0901388

[5] Wan XL, Yang ZB, Yang WR, Jiang SZ, Zhang GG, Johnston SL, Chi F. Toxicity of increasing aflatoxin B1 concentrations from contaminated corn with or without clay adsorbent supplementation in ducklings. Poultry Science. 2013;**92**:1244-1253. DOI: 10.3382/ps.2012-02748

[6] Kitya D, Bbosa GS, Mulogo E. Aflatoxin levels in common foods of south western Uganda: A risk factor to hepatocellular carcinoma. European Journal of Cancer Care. 2010;**19**:516-521. DOI: 10.1111/j.1365-2354.2009.01087.x

[7] Shirima CP, Kimanya ME, Routledge MN, Srey C, Kinabo JL, Humpf HU, Wild CP, Tu YK, Gong YY. A prospective study of growth and biomarkers of exposure to aflatoxin and fumonisin during early childhood in Tanzania. Environmental Health Perspectives. 2015;**123**:173-178. DOI: 10.1289/ehp.1408097

[8] Ezekiel CN, Bandyopadhyay R, Sulyok M, Warth B, Krska R. Fungal and bacterial metabolites in commercial poultry feed from Nigeria. Food Additives & Contaminants. Part A, Chemistry, Analysis, Control, Exposure & Risk Assessment. 2012;**29**:1288-1299. DOI: 10.1080/19440049.2012.688878

[9] Feddern V, Dors GC, Tavernari F, De C, Mazzuco H, Cunha AJ, Krabbe EL, Scheuermann GN. Aflatoxins importance on animal nutrition. In Aflatoxins - Recent advances and future prospects; Razzaghi-Abyaneh, M Ed., London: IntechOpen Limited; 2013. pp. 171-195

[10] Wu F, Khlangwiset P. Health economic impacts and cost-effectiveness of aflatoxin-reduction strategies in Africa: Case studies in biocontrol and post-harvest interventions. Food Additives & Contaminants. Part A, Chemistry, Analysis, Control, Exposure & Risk Assessment. 2010;**27**:496-509. DOI: 10.1080/19440040903437865

[11] Wu F, Guclu H. Aflatoxin regulations in a network of global maize trade. PLoS One. 2012;**7**:1-8

[12] Africa, P. for A. C. in PACA Strategy; 2013

[13] Lewis L, Onsongo M, Njapau H, Schurz-Rogers H, Luber G, Kieszak S, Nyamongo J, Backer L, Dahiye AM, Misore A, DeCock K, Rubin C. Aflatoxin contamination of commercial maize products during an outbreak of acute aflatoxicosis in eastern and Central Kenya. Environmental Health Perspectives. 2005;**113**:1763-1767. DOI: 10.1289/ehp.7998

[14] Asiki G, Seeley J, Srey C, Baisley K, Lightfoot T, Archileo K, Agol D, Abaasa A, Wakeham K, Routledge MN, Wild CP, Newton R, Gong YY. A pilot study to evaluate aflatoxin exposure in a rural Ugandan population. Tropical Medicine & International Health. 2014;**19**:592-599

[15] Kpodo KA, Bankole SA. Mycotoxin contamination in foods in West and Central Africa. In: Leslie JF, Bandyopadhyay R, Visconti A, editors. Mycotoxins. Detection Methods, Management, Public Heallth and Agricultural Trade. CABI International; 2008. pp. 103-116

[16] Ezekiel CN, Warth B, Ogara IM, Abia WA, Ezekiel VC, Atehnkeng J, Sulyok M, Turner PC, Tayo GO, Krska R, Bandyopadhyay R. Mycotoxin exposure in rural residents in northern Nigeria: A pilot study using multi-urinary biomarkers. Environment International. 2014;**66**:138-145. DOI: 10.1016/j.envint.2014.02.003

[17] Egal S, Hounsa A, Gong YY, Turner PC, Wild CP, Hall AJ, Hell K, Cardwell KF. Dietary exposure to aflatoxin from maize and groundnut in young children from Benin and Togo, West Africa. International Journal of Food Microbiology. 2005;**104**:215-224

[18] Okoth, S. Improving the Evidence Base on Aflatoxin Contamination and Exposure in Africa. CTA Working Paper 16/13. CTA and PACA. 2016; 1-113

[19] Gong YY, Cardwell K, Hounsa A, Egal S, Turner PC, Hall AJ, Wild CP. Dietary aflatoxin exposure and impaired growth in young children from Benin and Togo: Cross sectional study. BMJ. 2002;**325**:20-21

[20] Weaver M, Abbas H, Brewer M, Pruter L, Little N. Integration of biological control and transgenic insect protection for mitigation of mycotoxins in corn. Crop Protection. 2017; **98**:108-115. DOI: http://doi.org/10.1016/j.cropro.2017.03.020

[21] Blount WP. Tukey "X" disease. Turkeys. 1961;**9**:52-78

[22] Frazzoli C, Gherardi P, Saxena N, Belluzzi G, Mantovani A. The hotspot for (global) one health in primary food production: Aflatoxin M1 in dairy products. Frontiers in Public Health. 2017;**4**:1-11. DOI: 10.3389/fpubh.2016.00294

[23] Sundsmo A, Gwinner V, Nelson F, Othieno OR, Manyong V. Building an aflatoxin safe east African community technical policy paper 11. In: Five-Year Communication Strategy for Aflatoxin Safe East African Community. 2015

[24] PACA. PACA Begins Creation of Africa Aflatoxin Information Management System (Africa AIMS). Available online: http://www.aflatoxinpartnership.org/?q=node/335 [Accessed: Feb 5, 2017]

[25] World Food Program Connecting farmers to markets. Available online: https://www.wfp.org/purchase-progress/overview [Accessed: Feb 5, 2018]

[26] Fraser O. Regional workshop on combating aflatoxins in the maize value chains of Africa. In: Panel Discussion: Challenges and Opportunities for Aflatoxin Control by Value Chain Actors: Dar es Salam, Tanzania; 2017

[27] Nestle Grains Quality Improvement Project . Available online: https://www.nestle-cwa.com/en/media/newsandfeatures/grainsqualityimprovementproject

[28] Partnership for Aflatoxin Control in Africa Activities in Africa – Ghana. Available online: http://www.aflatoxinpartnership.org/?q=ghana [Accessed: May 16, 2018]

[29] IITA Aflasafe. Safer food in Africa. Available online: https://aflasafe.com/ [Accessed: Feb 5, 2018]

[30] Abt Associates. AgResults Evaluation Design: Nigeria Aflasafe Pilot; 2014

[31] AgResults Initiative Nigeria AflasafeTM Pilot. Available online: http://agresults.org/en/283/NigeriaAflasafePilot [Accessed: Feb 5, 2018]

[32] Pretty J, Toulmin C, Williams S. Sustainable intensification in African agriculture. International Journal of Agricultural Sustainability. 2011;**9**:5-24. DOI: 10.3763/ijas.2010.0583

[33] Carvajal-Campos A, Manizan AL, Tadrist S, Akaki DK, Koffi-Nevry R, Moore GG, Fapohunda SO, Bailly S, Montet D, Oswald IP, Lorber S, Brabet C, Puel O. Aspergillus korhogoensis, a novel aflatoxin producing species from the Côte d'Ivoire. Toxins (Basel). 2017;**9**:1-22. DOI: 10.3390/toxins9110353

[34] Kaaya AN, Warren HL, Kyamanywa S, Kyamuhangire W. The effect of delayed harvest on moisture content, insect damage, moulds and aflatoxin contamination of maize in Mayuge district of Uganda. Journal of the Science of Food and Agriculture. 2005;**85**:2595-2599. DOI: 10.1002/jsfa.2313

[35] Canavar O, Kaynak MA. Prevention of pre-harvest aflatoxin production and the effect of different harvest times on peanut (*Arachis hypogaea* L.) fatty acids. Food Additives & Contaminants: Part A. 2013;**30**:1807-1818

[36] Mehl HL, Cotty PJ. Variation in competitive ability among isolates of *Aspergillus flavus* from different vegetative compatibility groups during maize infection. Phytopathology. 2010;**100**:150-159. DOI: 10.1094/PHYTO-100-2-0150

[37] Guo B, Chen Z-Y, Lee RD, Scully BT. Drought stress and preharvest aflatoxin contamination in agricultural commodity: Genetics, genomics and proteomics. Journal of Integrative Plant Biology. 2008;**50**:1281-1291

[38] Brown RL, Menkir A, Chen ZY, Bhatnagar D, Yu J, Yao H, Cleveland TE. Breeding aflatoxin-resistant maize lines using recent advances in technologies–A review. Food Additives & Contaminants. Part A, Chemistry, Analysis, Control, Exposure & Risk Assessment. 2013;**30**:1382-1391. DOI: 10.1080/19440049.2013.812808

[39] ICRISAT. New study shows that groundnut immunity to aflatoxin could be within reach thanks to a double-defence approach. Available online: http://www.icrisat.org/groundnut-immunity-to-aflatoxin/ [Accessed: Feb 5, 2018]

[40] Njoroge SMC, Matumba L, Kanenga K, Siambi M, Waliyar F, Maruwo J, Monyo E. A case for regular aflatoxin monitoring in peanut butter in sub-Saharan Africa: Lessons from a 3-year survey in Zambia. Journal of Food Protection. 2016;**79**:795-800

[41] Matumba L, Monjerezi M, Khonga EB, Lakudzala DD. Aflatoxins in sorghum, sorghum malt and traditional opaque beer in southern Malawi. Food Control. 2011;**22**:266-268

[42] Akano DA, Atanda O. The present level of aflatoxin in Nigerian groundnut cake ("kuli-kuli"). Letters in Applied Microbiology. 1990;**10**:187-189

[43] Shephard GS. Aflatoxin and food safety: Recent African perspectives. Journal of Toxicology–Toxin Reviews. 2003;**22**:267-286

[44] Bullerman LB, Bianchini A. Stability of mycotoxins during food processing. International Journal of Food Microbiology. 2007;**119**:140-146. DOI: 10.1016/j.ijfoodmicro.2007.07.035

[45] Fandohan P, Zoumenou D, Hounhouigan DJ, Marasas WF, Wingfield MJ, Hell K. Fate of aflatoxins and fumonisins during the processing of maize into food products in Benin. International Journal of Food Microbiology. 2005;**98**:249-259. DOI: 10.1016/j.ijfoodmicro.2004.07.007

[46] Bailey GS, Price LR, Park DL, Hendricks JD. Effect of ammoniation of aflatoxin B1-contaminated cottonseed feedstock on the aflatoxin M1 content of cows' milk and hepatocarcinogenicity in the trout bioassay. Food and Chemical Toxicology. 1994;**32**:707-715

[47] Jaynes WF, Zartman RE. Aflatoxin toxicity reduction in feed by enhanced binding to surface-modified clay additives. Toxins (Basel). 2011;**3**:551-565

[48] Méndez-Albores JA, Arámbula-Villa G, Loarca-Piña MG, González-Hernández J, Castaño-Tostado E, Moreno-Martínezc E. Aflatoxins' fate during the nixtamalization of contaminated maize by two tortilla-making processes. Journal of Stored Products Research. 2004;**40**:87-94

[49] Herzallah S, Alshawabkeh K, Al Fataftah A. Aflatoxin decontamination of artificially contaminated feeds by sunlight, γ-radiation, and microwave heating. Journal of Applied Poultry Research. 2008;**17**:515-521. DOI: 10.3382/japr.2007-00107

Section 3

Aflatoxicosis and Control in Poultry

Chapter 7

Aflatoxins: Their Toxic Effect on Poultry and Recent Advances in Their Treatment

Yasir Allah Ditta, Saima Mahad and Umar Bacha

Additional information is available at the end of the chapter

http://dx.doi.org/10.5772/intechopen.80363

Abstract

About 25% of total agriculture products are contaminated with aflatoxins (AFs) and other mycotoxins in the world especially in Africa, Asia and Latin America, completely losing about 2–3% of food values and thus causing economic losses to farmers. The mycotoxin contaminations of food supply chain impact on human and animal health primarily, whereas production is the second major concern especially in developing countries. Aflatoxins (colorless to pale yellow colored crystals) are the most studied (>5000 research articles) group of mycotoxins. AFs impose major problems regarding health, growth, FCR (feed conversion ratio), etc. in the subtropical zone. In the agricultural commodities, the prevention of fungal contamination during plant growth, harvesting and storage seems to be the most effective and rational precautionary measures to avoid mycotoxins. Activated charcoal; aluminosilicates; polymers, such as polyvinyl pyrrolidones and cholestyramine; and yeast, yeast-based products, and humic acid have been studied extensively with promising but variable results. A live yeast, named Saccharomyces cerevisiae (*S. cerevisiae*), has also been observed to lighten the adverse effects of aflatoxicosis in poultry. These beneficial effects were later attributed to glucomannan, being derived from the cell wall of *S. cerevisiae*.

Keywords: aflatoxins, poultry, toxin binders

1. Background

Mycotoxins are known to affect human and animal health since 1370s BC. Ergotism or St. Anthony's fire is one of the oldest known mycotoxins. The mysterious deaths of archeologists are also considered due to the prevalence of ochratoxin A (OTA) in certain Egyptian tombs [1]. In 1673, the disease was linked to consumption of grains infected with ergot (sclerotia of

Claviceps purpurea) in France. An epidemic resulted in first ergotism control measures in 1770. In 1952, an outbreak of "moldy corn toxicosis" was caused by the consumption of mold contaminated corn-based feed for swine in southern USA [2]. In the early 1960s, over 100,000 turkey poults and 20,000 ducklings, pheasants and partridges poults in England died with clinical signs of liver necrosis and biliary hyperplasia. This incidence brought together world renowned scientists under the umbrella to resolve the puzzle related to turkey "X" disease [3, 4]. Brazilian peanuts used in formulating feeds for these domesticated animals were found to be heavily infected with aflatoxin B_1 (AFB_1) were found to be the main reason for this huge fatality after a series of analyses in England [3] and was named after *Aspergillus flavus* in 1962. A year later (in 1963), its complete structure was characterized by Prof. Buchi's team [1] and subsequently, aflatoxins (AFs) were further categorized as AFB and AFG because of blue and green fluorescence under UV light, respectively [3]. The most extensively publicized case came under the spotlight with an outbreak in humans in western India in October 1974 [5]. Unseasonal rainfall resulted in extensive mold production of extremely high AFs (6.3–15.6 mg/kg) in corn crops [6]. In 2004, several hundreds of Kenyans became severely ill and almost 125 casualties were reported during an acute aflatoxicosis outbreak [7]. Since the identification of Aflatoxins (AFs) in 1965, the momentum of scientific paper publication toward mycotoxin is an increasing trend where 16,821 papers are recorded in Scopus and is an indicative of its importance [8].

2. Mycotoxins

Mycotoxins (MW $\sim$ 700 Da) are secondary metabolites produced by mycelial filamentous structures, specifically called molds [4, 9, 10]. Aspergillus, Penicillium and Fusarium species are responsible for the production of most prevalent mycotoxins, i.e. AFs, ochratoxin, zearalenone, deoxynivalenole, trichothecene-2, etc. [11]. Cereals are more prone to mycotoxins contamination by fungal growth on plants in fields or fungi growing saprophytically during storage. Not all fungal growth results in mycotoxins production (e.g. penicillin, is widely used an antibiotic) or the detection of fungi implies necessarily the presence of mycotoxins [12, 13]. All the secondary metabolites from molds do not impose toxic effects [4].

In response to the environment, five different mechanisms are involved in the production of mycotoxins viz. secondary fungal metabolism, bioconversion of plant compounds (dicoumarol), defense mechanism of plants to fungal aggression and plant-fungus associations [9]. Among the environmental conditions, agronomic practices including harvesting technology as well as the health status of the plant are the most approachable factors for fungal contamination in plants and ultimately mycotoxin production. Humans and animals can be exposed to mycotoxins by various routes like ingestion, aerosol and placental routes [14], which may lead to different fatal consequences as these toxins can be carcinogenic, neurotoxic and immunotoxic, mutagenic, teratogenic, esterogenic and/or hepatotoxic [15]. The severity of health effects posed by mycotoxins depends on species, sex, age, nutritional status, etc. [16]. AFs, OTA and possibly fumonisin B_1 (FB_1) have been classified as being carcinogenic [9]. All countries with mycotoxins regulations should have at least regulatory limits for AFB_1 or the sum of AFB_1, AFB_2, AFG_1, and AFG_2 in foods and/or feeds [11]. Mycotoxins exposure includes both pure mycotoxins and also masked mycotoxins which are formed when plants protect themselves by conjugating mycotoxins to biopolymers [8].

3. Factors affecting mycotoxin production

Cereals and their products are susceptible to fungal invasion that may be accompanied by mycotoxin production [17]. Approximately 25–40% of cereals produced worldwide are directly or indirectly contaminated with mycotoxins especially AFs with annual losses of around 1 billion MT of food products [9, 18]. *A. flavus* and *A. parasiticus* are responsible for producing AF during storage particularly in hot and humid countries in the tropics as compared to those in the temperate regions of the world [9, 19].

A. flavus is commonly found in energy rich concentrates (corn, rice etc.) and protein rich concentrates (peanuts, cottonseed etc.) but are not commonly found in tree nuts. *A. parasiticus* occurrence in South East Asia is rare and has the same hosts as those of *A. flavus* [20]. *A. flavus* is generally responsible for AFB_1 and AFB_2 production, whereas *A. parasiticus* produces AFB_1, B_2, G_1 and G_2 [3]. AFB_1 ranges 77% of total AFs as major contaminant in cereals [21]. In the grains, the germ is the main site for *Aspergillus* sp. development which leads to greater potential of AF accumulation [22].

The on-going global warming is going to be an alarming condition for the aflatoxins contamination [8]. Williams et al. [23] observed that improperly dried stored food is commonly invaded by fungus (Aspergillus sp.) in areas within latitude 40°N and 40°S of the equator with temperatures that range between 24 and 35°C and moisture content >7% (10% with ventilation). About 4.5 billion people are chronically exposed to AFs in developing countries. Tropical and sub-tropical regions have favorable environment for AFs production as compared to temperate region [19, 24].

4. Mycotoxin occurrence

Binder et al. [11] found low concentrations of Deoxynivalenol, T-2 toxin and Zearalenone as major contaminants in European (temperate areas) feed samples while AFs, DON, FUM and ZON tended to be dominant in Asia and Pacific (tropical areas) significantly. Elzupir et al. [25] found a total of 64.29% animal feed (130.63 μg/kg) and 87.50% manufactured animal rations (54.41–579.87 μg/kg) followed by 69.32% groundnut samples (4.07–79.85 μg/kg) contaminated with AFs in Khartoum State of Sudan. Summer was found to be the most favorable for AFs growth (78.95% samples) followed by autumn (66.67% samples) and winter season (43.37% samples). AFB_1 was found the most common contaminant followed by AFG_1, AFB_2 and AFG_2.

Shareef [26] found AFs to be most prevalent mycotoxins group (91.1%) with average concentration of 179.1 μg/kg followed by ochratoxins (127 μg/kg) during a two-year survey (2005–2007) on different poultry feed samples in Pakistan. Anjum et al. [27] found AFB_2 (10.80 ± 2.16 to 39.20 ± 3.67 μg/kg) in layer and broiler starter rations from ten different commercial feed mills in Punjab, Pakistan. Among them, 40% of samples were contained AFB_2 at levels above 20 μg/kg (maximum tolerable levels for poultry). Bokhari [29] found 26.1% samples (seeds, oilseeds, spices, milk and milk products) contaminated with AFs principally poultry feed, cereal grains and oil seeds with AFB_1 found as the most frequent contaminant especially in corn grains.

Luttfullah and Hussain [29] found maximum incidence rate of AFs in walnuts with shell (40%), walnuts without shell (70%) and in peanuts with shell (40%) during a survey in Khyber Pakhtun and northern areas of Pakistan. Lutfullah and Arshad [30] found highest AFs incidence rate in corn (40%), sorghum (30%) and rice (25%) from different retail shops and local markets of different location in Pakistan. In Pakistan, *A. flavus* contamination occurs at the highest incidence rate, being responsible for the production of AFB_1 in the corn in Swat valley [31].

Borutova et al. [32] found a positive correlation between AFB_1 and AFB_2 prevalence on different feedstuffs i.e. corn, wheat, soybean meal, corn gluten meal, dried distiller grains, etc. in Asian-Oceania region in 2010 and concluded that the occurrence of single mycotoxins in any of the feedstuffs is rare. Mardani et al. [33] did not find via High Performance Liquid Chromatography (HPLC) any of the AFs at detectable levels in food samples from Kaskinen in Iran except for one sample that contained AFB_1 (0.64 μg/kg). Basaran and Ozcan (2009) concluded AFB_1 to be the most abundant in concentration (0.2–36.81 μg/kg) followed by four samples containing AFG_1 (0.6–20.2 μg/kg) among 217 samples of hazelnuts, pistachio nuts and peanuts in the Turkey. About 87.09% of total samples were very low in AFB_1.

5. Chemical nature and structural illustration

Due to recent advances in technology, modern methods and budding interests, more than 300–500 mycotoxins have been discovered and characterized. Mycotoxins have very special chemical configurations [11, 18, 34]. However, only a relatively small number of toxins are of relevance in feed milling [11]. The AFs are difurocoumaro-lactones (difurocoumarin derivatives) in structure. These chemical structures comprise of a difuran ring with complex coumarin nucleus with a pentenone ring (in AFB and AFM)/a six membered lactone ring (AFG). The four compounds viz. AFB_1, B_2, G_1 and G_2 (**Figure 1**) can be differentiated by fluorescence under ultraviolet illumination (B = blue, G = green) [3]. AFs are indistinctly soluble in H_2O and hydrocarbons, soluble in methanol, acetone and chloroform and insoluble in non-polar solvents. They appear to be unstable in air and light. These toxins are decomposed at their respective melting points which range between 237°C (G) and 299°C (M_1) but not destroyed under normal cooking conditions. Rather these can be completely denatured by autoclaving in the presence of NH_3 or by treatment with bleach [35].

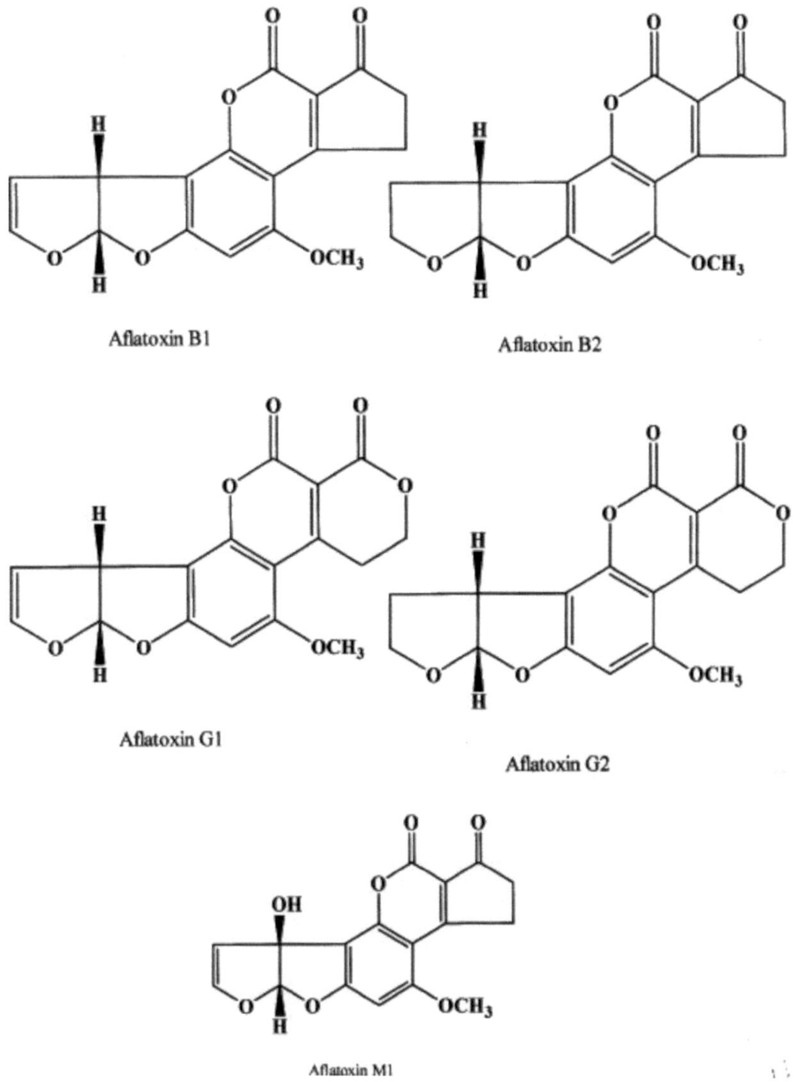

Figure 1. The chemical structure of aflatoxins [19].

6. Levels of toxin production

According to Wayne [43], the amount of toxins produced depends on different factors that can be physical, chemical or biological. Physical factors include moisture, relative humidity, temperature and mechanical damage, while chemical factors include CO_2, O_2, substrate composition, pesticide and fungicide. Plant variety, stress (harsh weather), insects, and spore concentration collectively are biological factors that may affect toxin production.

Temperature, water activity (a_w), oxygen and pH [1, 27, 36–39] play vital role in the production of mycotoxins by fungi. The a_w range should be between 0.61 and 0.91 as most of storage fungi grow at aw <0.75. The ideal temperature for AFs production by *A. flavus* and *A. parasiticus* ranges between 12 and 41°C with optimum production occurring at 25–32°C. But the AF synthesis increases by temperature >27°C, humidity >62% and moisture >14% [3]. Relative to AFG_1, AFB_1 production is stimulated by higher temperature [40]. Optimal production of AFB_1 occurs between 24 and 28°C, whereas 23°C is optimal for AFG_1 production. Low temperature (8–10°C) induces the production of equal amounts of AFB and AFG. However, total AFs production is suppressed with more time is required [3]. At higher a_w, fungi compete with bacteria as food spoilers [17]. Moreover, *Aspergillus* can tolerate lower aw than *Fusarium* [41]. Initially, fungal growth in grains produces adequate metabolic water for further expansion and mycotoxins production [42]. Oxygen is an essential factor for the fungal growth and its growth is restricted at less than 1% oxygen [17].

The broken grains (by insects and birds) are often more susceptible to mycotoxins production. The grains with "musty" odor should be suspected and analyzed for mycotoxins [42]. Aflatoxins contamination is directly influenced by insects' attack to plants and is probably dominated by drought and high temperature [43]. These predisposing conditions allow "hot spots" to occur in stored grains. In severely affected crop of corn, the individual kernel may contain AFs as high as 400,000 μg/kg AFs [42].

The accrual of mycotoxins in the grains before and after harvest largely reflects the prevailing climatic conditions. For example, *Fusarium* toxins are produced in cereals with high moisture content during harvest, whereas pre-harvest AF contamination of crops like peanuts and maize is linked with high temperatures, insect damage and prolonged drought conditions [43].

Fungal geneticists have unraveled the pathways and genes for the synthesis and regulation of mycotoxins production, especially AFs and trichothecenes [37, 44], which assist in the breeding of plants resistant to toxin accumulation [45]. The transgenic Bt corn contains a gene isolated from the soil bacterium *Bacillus thuringiensis,* which encodes for a protein, being toxic to common lepidopteran corn pests. These hybrids offer a new tool for mycotoxins management as insect damage is often a major factor in facilitating toxigenic fungal infection of crops [46].

7. Toxicity of aflatoxins

AF (AFB_1, G_1, B_2 and G_2) concentration, duration of dietary exposure, species, sex, breed, age and health status of animals are different factors that affect toxicity [42, 47]. Young animals are less resistant than older one presumably due to the lack of well-developed hepatic enzymatic systems required to degrade the toxins depending upon the specie [48]. Guinea-pig, duckling and rabbit represent a "fast metabolizing group" actually capable of handling LD50 dose in <12 minutes. Sheep, pig, mouse and chick fall into "intermediate group" metabolizing LD50 dose in few hours [49]. Currently, rat is the only example of a "slow metabolizing group" in which LD50 dose would probably disappear from the liver over a period of days (Hu et al.,

2011). AFB_1 is classified by IARC [35], as a highly toxic compound (LD50, 1–50 mg/kg body weight) among most species, although it is extremely toxic (LD50 < 1 mg/kg) for some species such as cats, ducklings and rainbow trouts [3].

Ducklings followed by turkey poults, broilers and laying hens are the most sensitive species to AFs as these showed 100% mortality at 1 mg/kg AFB_1. Moreover, 0.11–0.2 mg/kg AFB_1 decreased 230 and 163 g/bird feed intake and weight, approximately from 0 to 14 days of age, respectively [50]. Goslings, quails and pheasants are ranked at intermediate position regarding sensitivity while chickens appear to be the highly resistant. Ducklings are 5–15 times more sensitive than laying hens, but among layers, certain strains may be as much as 3 times more sensitive than others [38]. Broilers are more susceptible to AF than layers [36, 51]. Aflatoxin-contaminated feed affect almost all systems in the body are affected, i.e. interference in bone metabolism resulting decreased bone strength, reduction in bone diameter, decrease in dressed weight and breast yield etc. [52].

8. Mode of action of aflatoxins

AFs are toxic to poultry at <1 mg/kg with liver as main target organ as the relative liver weight is altered by low levels of AFs [53, 54]. Respiratory exposure to AFB_1 contaminated dust has been allied with increased incidence levels of tumor along the respiratory tract of animals and humans [3]. The AFs molecules are subjected through complex metabolic processes of different cytochrome P450 dependent pathways (bio-activation or detoxification processes) [55].

The carcinogenic and mutagenic effects of AFB_1 [4], AFG_1 and AFM_1 occur after metabolic activation by microsomal mixed function oxidase system [3, 56]. AFs bind to both RNA and DNA and blocks transcription [17]. In the liver, cytochrome P450 activates AFB_1 (pro-carcinogens) to form AFB_1–8, 9-exo-epoxide (catalyzed by CYP3A4 leading to the formation of AFQ_1) and endo-epoxide (catalyzed by CYP1A2) at 8, 9 position of the terminal furan ring and its subsequent covalent binding to nucleic acid but only exo-epoxide that is highly unstable binds with DNA resulting in the formation of 8,9-dihydro-8-(N7-guanyl)-9-hydro-AFB_1 (AFB_1-N7-Gua) adduct [18, 56, 57]. Toxin interaction with DNA and some enzymes to alter *p53* gene results in GC to TA transversion, which results in mutagenic properties. This transversion is capable of binding to lysine in serum albumin [58] and also inhibits different activities on biological molecules e.g. synthesis of DNA adducts and conjugation with glutathione, and blocks of ribosomal translocase and RNA polymerase (inhibiting protein synthesis) and essential enzymes [59]. The RNA and DNA syntheses were inhibited in rats fed feed contaminated with 5 mg/kg AFs of over six weeks period [4]. AFB1-epoxide can covalently bind to different proteins which in turn, may affect structural and enzymatic protein function [3]. The structure of interaction between base pairs in DNA helix is determined by binding of exo-epoxide with guanine [60, 61]. The metabolites (AFQ_1, AFM_1 and AFP_1) of AFB_1 and other naturally occurring AFs such as AFG_1, B_2 and G_2, are weaker for epoxide formation, thus they have less carcinogenic and toxic properties than AFB_1.

In liver cells, cytoplasmic reductase and microsomal mixed-function oxidase system metabolize AFB_1 to aflatoxicol and aflatoxins M_1, Q_1, P_1 and B_1-epoxide (the most toxic and carcinogenic derivative), which are less toxic than AFB1. These are further conjugate with other molecules and rapidly eliminated from the body [3]. The metabolites (AFQ_1, AFM_1 and AFP_1) being formed from AFB_1 and other naturally occurring AFs e.g. G_1, B_2 and G_2 are weaker for epoxidation, thus possess less carcinogenic and toxic properties than AFB_1. The AFM_1, AFQ_1 and AFP_1 are secreted as metabolites of AFB_1 in the urine and can be used as biomarkers [62].

9. Absorption of aflatoxins in small intestine

Aflatoxins are liposoluble compounds that are readily absorbed at the site of exposure (usually gastrointestinal tract) into the blood stream to liver where they are metabolized in the microsomal system to active or detoxified metabolites [63]. AFB_1 may occur as free or unconjugated forms of primary metabolites. Water soluble conjugate metabolites bound covalently with cellular macromolecules and degradation/metabolic products of AFB_1 adducts. These conjugates of AFB_1 metabolites are excreted in the bile and consequently eliminated through feces. Water soluble conjugates and degradation or metabolic products of AFB_1 macromolecule adducts and unconjugated AFB_1 metabolites are excreted into general circulatory blood system. This results the systemic distribution of AFB_1 to eggs or milk and body tissues [3].

AFs are known to alter the synthesis, absorption, and transport of lipids to extra-hepatic tissues. Liver fatty acid composition is drastically altered among birds with aflatoxicosis [43]. AFB1-8, 9-epoxide (formed by action of cytochrome P450 on AFB_1) may cause significant increase in hepatic lipid peroxide level. Lipid peroxidation initiates to affect membrane integrity negatively; membrane bound enzyme activities which lead to cell lysis. The oxidative damage of cell/tissue occurs when the concentration of reactive oxygen species ($O_2\cdot$, H_2O_2, and $OH\cdot$) predominates the antioxidant capability of cells. This may be the consequence of significant decrease in non-enzymatic antioxidants (e.g. glutathione, vitamin E, and vitamin C) and enzymatic antioxidants (e.g. catalase, glutathione peroxidase, superoxide dismutase). Superoxide dismutase shields cells from oxidative damage by metabolizing free radical superoxide ($O_2\cdot$) to H_2O_2 and $O_2\cdot$. The metabolically produced H_2O_2 can then be decomposed enzymatically with glutathione peroxidase (GSH-Px) and catalase. Glutathione peroxidase not only decomposes H_2O_2 but also can interact with lipid peroxidation. Reduced protein biosynthesis may be responsible for the decline in enzyme activities. Significantly lower glutathione peroxidase levels further intensify the toxic effects of AFs [24]. AFs promote free radical formation thus causing liver peroxidation which in turn results in antioxidant depletion, oxidative stress and apoptosis. All of these contribute to the development of malabsorption [64].

The metabolites such as AFB_1-N_7-Gua, AFM_1, AFB_1-mercapturic acid and serum AFs-albumin are also considered as AF biomarkers [65]. AFs show specific selection for guanine bases with a guanine or cytosine at the 5′ base causing G → T transversion [66]. Puisieux et al. [67] showed that the guanine at the third position of codon 249 of the *p53* gene (a known mutational hotspot in HCC (hepatocellular carcinoma) was the site of modification by AFB_1 (in human hepatocytes, about three folds mutations at the third base of codon 249) but neighboring guanines (247, 248 and 250) were also modified. About 20% of total AFB_1 ingested remain in the body after a period of one week with a half-life in the plasma of 36.5 minutes, whereas M_1 is almost excreted via urine within 48 hours [68]. Because there is a half-life of 20 days in serum albumin, the AFB_1-albumin adduct can be used as an AF biomarker to check the chronic exposure within 1–2 months and is considered as an independent factor for advanced liver diseases in HCV-infected patients. The adduction levels of AFs with albumin by covalent bonding in the peripheral blood reflect AF exposure 2–3 months earlier depending on albumin half-life [66].

10. Effect of aflatoxins on enzymes

A marked decrease in digestive enzymes (pancreatic ribonuclease, amylase, trypsin and lipase), hypocarotenoidaemia, steatorrhea and bile salts can be observed during aflatoxicosis in poultry. Protein requirements for growth were increased during aflatoxicosis which can be alleviated by dietary methionine fortification [43]. Fernandez et al. [69] conducted trials to investigate the hematological and serological changes on broilers from 21 to 42 days of age with oral administration of 2500 μg/kg AFB_1. It was found that hematological (red blood cell, hemoglobin, leucocytes, eosinophils and basophils) and serological (serum protein, aspartate aminotransferase, alanine aminotransferase, urea, creatinine) parameters remained unchanged but caused hepatic and renal lesions which matches the findings of Bianchi et al. [39]. AFs are known to reduce protein synthesis that may lead to decreased blood protein levels. The AFs intoxications have been reported to decrease total protein, cholesterol, triglyceride and glucose levels significantly [70].

11. "Carry-over" of aflatoxins

Mycotoxins including Aflatoxins are metabolized in the gastrointestinal tract, liver or kidneys according to their chemical structure. Their transfer to poultry meat and eggs leads to undesirable effects on human health [18]. Agag [3] examined the *"carry-over"* of AFB_1 from layer feed to eggs was examined in laying hens at dietary levels of 100–400 μg/kg AFB1. This resulted in 0.2 to 3.3 μg/kg in eggs, and AFs ratios in feeds and tissues found to be are very low ranging from 500:1 to 14,000:1 excluding the liver, particularly when compared with milk (70:1). On the other hand, Zaghini et al. [55] showed no measurable residual AFB_1 or its metabolites in eggs. These contrasting findings may be ascribed to mannan oligosaccharides in naturally AFs contaminated feeds at different levels of toxicity [55].

In broilers and layer birds, the AFB_1 residues have been reported to vary from no detection to 3.0 μg/kg in liver in birds fed 250–3310 μg/kg AFB_1 over certain periods [71]. Fowler et al. [72] found no significant increase in AFs residues in liver until the 1800 μg/kg AF contaminated feed was fortified with AF at a concentration of 1200 μg/kg with no clay used as a binding agent. Younger birds were found to have significant increase in liver residues than those in non-exposed birds. Moreover, birds 3rd weeks of age that received 1800 μg/kg AFs were found to have detectable levels of AFB_1 in the liver.

12. Immunosuppression

Aflatoxins intoxications suppress immunoglobulins (IgM, IgG and IgA) and enhance susceptibility of birds to parasitic, viral and bacterial infections. At 0.5 to 1 mg/kg Aflatoxins, these interfere with B and T-lymphocytes functioning [73], apparent alteration of splenic functioning, atrophy of bursa of Fabricius [74], suppresses cell mediated immune response, phagocytosis, and complement system as well as interferon production. Moreover, hematopoietic suppression and anemia have been observed by decrease in RBCs, packed cell volume and hemoglobin [75–78].

AFs decrease total serum proteins due to a reduction in α, β and γ globulins, with IgG being more sensitive than IgM [79] which may cause substantial suppression of acquired immunity from vaccination programs in some disease models. The Low levels of AFB_1 appears to affect the vaccinal immunity negatively and may enhance the occurrence of diseases such as Marek's disease, IBD virus, congenitally acquired salmonellosis and duodenal and cecal coccidiosis, etc. even in properly vaccinated flocks [80]. The failure of vaccines is correlated to the immunotoxic effect of toxins which compromise for immune function of birds by decreasing cell-mediated immunity and inducing an inflammatory response [81]. Decrease chemotactic ability of leucocytes, impaired heterophils phagocytosis [3] and cellular and serum factors required for optimal phagocytosis can be observed in aflatoxicated chickens. Although dietary AFs depress thrombocyte counts, no effect on their phagocytic activity has been observed [82].

13. Safe level of aflatoxins and detoxification

Due to synergistic effect of Aflatoxin B_1 and hepatitis B exposure, there are no specific safe levels for aflatoxin regarding resistance/tolerance to AFs. Ideally, there should be zero level for AFs in feed [83]. The Food and Drug Administration and European Union have established 20 μg/kg and 10 μg/kg AFs as maximum level for poultry, respectively. Based on feeds available, AF contaminated feeds should be fed at lowest possible level and for the shortest period of time [84]. The production of AFs can be controlled by maintaining physical integrity of cereal grains, drying and use of anti-fungal especially propionic acid to inhibits molds growth by decreasing pH and ATP formation through electron transport pathway. UV, X-rays or microwave irradiation and dilution of contaminated feed with AF free feed is also one of the methods to dilute the concentration of AFs [9]. However, AFB_1 contamination of feed is practically unavoidable universally [85]. Mycotoxins decontamination refers to methods by which these metabolites are removed or neutralized in contaminated feed, while mycotoxins detoxification refers to methods by which the toxic properties of the mycotoxins are eliminated [86]. Since early 1990s, studies on mycotoxin adsorbents have yielded success but high inclusion rates and potential interactions with dietary nutrients are causes for concern [87]. Numerous strategies for the detoxification and inactivation of mycotoxins in feed have been tested but most of these are ineffective or impractical [22]. Dietary fortification with methionine, selenium, vitamins, plant and herbal formulations, etc. may detoxify the adverse effects of AFs by glutathione systems which contain cysteine (derivatives of methionine) in broilers [43, 86]. Approaches to detoxify contaminated grain and finished feed can be physical, chemical and biological treatments [88].

14. Physical and chemical methods

Thermal inactivation, cleaning of the kernel surface, and hence the removal of highly contaminated particulate matter, have proven effective in reducing moderate mycotoxins contamination of feed [43, 89]. However, it seems quite laborious to remove highly contaminated feedstuffs. On the other hand, a lot of chemicals e.g. acids (sulfuric acid, hydrochloric acid, phosphoric acid, benzoic acid, citric acid, acetic acid), alkaline compounds (ammonia, sodium bicarbonate, sodium hydroxide, potassium hydroxide, calcium hydroxide, caustic soda), salts (acetate ammonium, sodium bisulfite, sodium hydrosulfite, sodium chloride, sodium sulfate), oxidants (H_2O_2, sodium hypochlorite, ozone), reducing agents (bisulfites), chlorinated agents and formaldehyde, etc., are being used for the degradation of mycotoxins in feed [90]. These methods are inefficient but comparatively expensive. Ammoniation has been demonstrated to reduce AFs levels but not accepted in the United States [91].

High level dosages of methyl bromide, ethylene dibromide, propane/propene ethylene oxide, sulfur dioxide, phosphine propionic, acetic and isobutyric acids show fungicidal activity. However, these chemicals lower nutritional quality and are corrosive on human and animal tissues [92]. Therefore, the use of these chemicals is discouraged. Several related patents involving the use of ozone in agricultural products decontamination are found. This decontamination method involves placing the agricultural products in a treatment chamber, generating ozone in the vicinity of chamber, supplying ozone to the product through continuous flow and exposing the agricultural product to ozone, which then reacts with the toxins and/or microorganisms.

There are different types of adsorbents, which can be used for the detoxification of AFs in the feed. The use of activated carbon for the detoxification of mycotoxins can also be another option but different activated charcoals have less/no effect against mycotoxins, which show their unspecified adsorbent nature. Moreover, certain essential nutrients are also adsorbed when at higher concentration in as compared to mycotoxins [93].

The most applied method for protecting animals against mycotoxicoses is the utilization of adsorbents in the feed, aimed at binding mycotoxins efficiently in the gastrointestinal tract, thus limiting or at best preventing the toxins from being absorbed by the body thereby, preventing their toxic effects and "carry over" of the toxins to animal products [89]. Selected adsorbents added to AFs-contaminated feeds as feed additives can sequester AFs during the digestive process, allowing the mycotoxins to pass harmlessly through the gastrointestinal tract of animal [94]. This is one of the more effective and practical approaches to address the problem of AFs.

The degree of adsorption capacities may vary (0–87%) among various mineral clay materials [95], and very few are actually used commercially. These considered as good absorbents include bentonites, zeolites and aluminosilicates. Studies have shown that sodium aluminosilicates, HSCAS (hydrated sodium calcium aluminosilicates) and sodium bentonites adsorb AFs [96] with adsorption potential of bentonites varying from 17 to 36%. A major advantage of these adsorbents is that they are relatively inexpensive and safe and can be easily incorporated in animal feeds [97].

Mineral adsorbents based on zeolites, silicates and phyllosilicates show different abilities to bind AFs. These possess active sites within interlayer channels at the basal planes on the surfaces or within pores, and at the edges of particles [98]. Bentonites are white, light weight and originate from volcanic ash comprising mainly of montmorillonite, the main constituent of bentonites. These are composed mostly of salts of Na, K, Ca of hydrated aluminosilicates and occasionally Fe, Mg, Zn, Ni, etc. but the composition varies from one deposit to another because of interchangeable mono and divalent ions e.g. Na^+, K^+, Ca^{+2}, and Mg^{+2}. So they can be classified as Ca, Mg, K or Na bentonites [86]. They have a layered microstructure, which allows AFs to bind at multiple sites including edges and basal surfaces especially at the interlayer region for adsorption [99, 100].

Zeolites possess strong colloidal properties to absorb water rapidly resulting in swelling and manifold increase in volume, giving rise to a thixotropic gelatinous substance [101, 102]. Hydration of the exchangeable cations creates a hydrophilic environment in the interlayer of montmorillonite, which influence the adsorption of different organic molecules, including mycotoxins on zeolite and montmorillonite particles [103]. The surfaces of zeolites derived HSCAS, attract polar functional groups of AFs, thus inhibit their absorption [93, 104] but is less effective against other mycotoxins. Zeolites selectively retain or release calcium during its passage through digestive system. Zeolites can absorb nitrogen of some amino acids and reduce the energy required for meat production. Zeolites suppress phosphorus utilization by forming indigestible compound with phosphorus through its aluminosilicate component [105]. Supplementation of HSCAS at the rate of 1.0% seems to diminish significantly, the adverse effects of AFs in young animals [93] as these have a high negative charge and are balanced by cations of such metals as magnesium, potassium and sodium located in the cavities, and therefore do not react with food/feed ingredients and act as inert material due to their neutral pH or slightly alkaline nature [106].

Aluminosilicates are also used at a level up to 2% as "anti-caking" agents but a several disadvantages have been observed including the impairment of minerals utilization and having a narrow range of binding efficacy [93]. Bentonites minerals can influence Ca-metabolism and bind nitrogenous cations such as NH_4^+. These are found to be effective for the adsorption of AFB_1 and T-2 toxin but not for zearalenone. Kececi et al. [107] determined decrease in calcium and phosphorus levels by AFs (2.5 mg/kg) for 21 days. Southern et al. [108] did not find any adverse effect on the growth and tibial mineral concentrations in chicks fed nutrient-deficient diets. Mineral clays reduce utilization of minerals including manganese, zinc, magnesium [109], chloride [95], copper and sodium [110]. Solís-Cruz et al. [111] conducted an *in vitro* study to evaluate the adsorption capacity of Chitosan (CHI), and three cellulosic polymers (Hydroxy propyl methyl cellulose, Sodium Carboxy methyl cellulose, and Microcrystalline Cellulose), on six mycotoxins (AFB_1; FUB_1; OTA; T-2; DON; and, ZEA) for poultry. All four cellulosic polymers showed significant ($p < 0.05$) binding activity against mycotoxins as compared to control with non-treated group. However Hydroxy propyl methyl cellulose, Sodium Carboxy methyl cellulose, and Microcrystalline Cellulose showed better adsorbent capacity for all mycotoxins when compared with Cholistan.

15. Biological methods

Various bacterial, yeast and fungal species are able to degrade/remove mycotoxins and also can restrict fungal growth. This includes the use of *Bacillus subtilis*, NK-330 and NK-C-3 that effectively inhibit the fungus growth and AFs production [92]. The application of micro-organisms e.g. *Corynebacterium rubrum* for bio-transformation of mycotoxins into less toxic metabolites is another option [9]. These micro-organisms act in intestinal tract of animals prior to absorption of mycotoxins but the concerned toxicity of products by enzymatic degradation and undesired effects of fermentation with non-native micro-organisms on food quality is yet to be investigated completely.

Saccharomyces cerevisiae and lactic acid bacteria (LAB) i.e. propionibacteria, bifidobacteria and *lactobacillus rhamnosus* strongly bind to their cell wall constituents mycotoxins without deleterious effects on animal health [9, 85, 93, 112]. Most yeast strains bind more than 15% (w/w) AFB_1, which is highly strain specific by *S. cerevisiae* [112] and LAB for mycotoxins detoxification [113]. Generally, *S. cerevisiae* shows very low adhesion to the intestines [114], as opposed to LAB that show considerable adhesion to intestinal cells [115]. Coallier-Ascah and Idziak [116] and Thyagaraja and Hosono [117] found LAB to be inefficient binders of AFB_1 due to the strains used, which may also depend on initial concentration of AFs [118]. Haskard et al. [119] showed that cell wall of *L. rhamnosus* has the ability to bind AFs predominantly to carbohydrates and to some extent, protein components that which is unaffected by pH of GI tract. The outer part of cell wall (26–32%) of *S. cerevisiae* contains a structure called glucomannan, which binds against mycotoxins [9]. The yeast cell wall comprises of 30–60% polysaccharides (β-glucan and mannan sugar polymers), 15–30% protein, 5–20% lipids and a small amount of chitin. Mainly, it contains 15–30% β-glucan and 15–30% MOS. Lahtinen et al. [120] found that peptidoglycans might be the most likely carbohydrate involved in the AFB_1 binding process [121]. Kusumaningtyas et al. [122] used *S. cerevisiae*, *Rhizopus oligosporus* and their combination for detoxifying AFB_1 in the chicken feed.

The supplementation of whole yeast and only yeast cell wall rather [53, 112, 123] have shown a reduction in mycotoxins toxicities, indicating possible stability of the yeast-mycotoxins complex along the gastrointestinal tract. The cell wall represents about 30% of total weight of yeast cell [112]. Glucomannan is a bi-layered structure that consists of a network of β-1,3 glucan with β-1,6 glucan side chains. This network is in turn attached to highly glycosylated mannoproteins. The proteins and glucans provide numerous easily accessible binding sites with different binding mechanisms such as Van Der Waals bonds, hydrogen bonding, ionic or hydrophobic interactions [93, 112, 124, 125]. Yeast glucomannan showed markedly high binding ability with AFs *in vitro* (75–90%) and *in vivo* [126, 127]. The carbohydrate fractions of cell wall may represent 90% of mannoproteins. MOS constitute approximately 50% of total carbohydrates [112]. The effect of 500 g of glucomannan is comparable with that of 8 Kg of clay for mycotoxins bindings [9].

16. Conclusion

Feed contamination by fungi can be a predicament for feed security. Under the current condition of temperature, humidity and global warming, the occurrence of mycotoxins including aflatoxins has become overbearing. There is a need for more research on multiple effects of mycotoxins, their trans-conversions and masked mycotoxins. New insights on the development of mycotoxins resistant seed varieties are need which could decrease the damage to grains in fields and during storage and thus could decrease the health risks and financial losses. The advances in Activated charcoal, aluminosilicates; polymers, such as polyvinyl pyrrolidones and cholestyramine, yeast, yeast based products and enzymatic deactivation have been quite successful to decrease the harmful effects of mycotoxins.

Author details

Yasir Allah Ditta[1]*, Saima Mahad[1] and Umar Bacha[2]

*Address all correspondence to: yasirad@uvas.edu.pk

1 Department of Animal Nutrition, University of Veterinary and Animal Sciences, Lahore, Pakistan

2 University of Management and Technology, Lahore, Pakistan

References

[1] Asoa T, Buchi G, Abdel-Kader MM, Chang SB, Wick EL, Wogan GN. Aflatoxins B and G. Journal of the American Chemical Society. 1963;**85**:1706-1707

[2] Sean PA. Mycotoxins and indoor molds. Indoor Environment Connections. 2002;**3**(4):14-24

[3] Agag BI. Mycotoxins in foods and feeds. 1-Aflatoxins. Assiut University Bulletin for Environmental Researches. 2004;**7**(1):173-206

[4] Hussein HS, Brasel JM. Toxicity, metabolism, and impact of mycotoxins on humans and animals. Toxicology. 2001;**167**(2):101-134. ISSN: 0300-483X. DOI: 10.1016/S0300-483X(01)00471-1. URL: http://www.sciencedirect.com/science /article/pii/S0300483 X01004711

[5] Reddy BN, Raghavender CR. Outbreaks of aflatoxicoses in India. African Journal of Food Agriculture Nutrition and Development. 2007;**7**:5

[6] Robens FJ, Richard JL. Aflatoxins in animal and human health. Reviews of Environmental Contamination and Toxicology. 1992;**127**:70-94

[7] Wu F, Clare M, Marites T, Yan L. The Health economics of aflatoxin: Global burden of disease. Facilitated by IFPRI. Working paper 4. 2011

[8] Liew W-P-P, Mohd-Redzwan S. Mycotoxin: Its impact on gut health and microbiota. Frontiers in Cellular and Infection Microbiology. 2018;**8**:60. DOI: 10.3389/fcimb.2018.00060

[9] Alexandros Y, Jean PJ. Mycotoxins in feeds and their fate in animals. Asian-Australasian Journal of Animal Sciences. 2002;**51**:81-99

[10] Dewegowda G, Raju MVLN, Swamy HVLN. Mycotoxins: Novel solutions for their conteraction. Feedstuffs. 1998;**7**(12):15

[11] Binder EM, Tan LM, Chin LJ, Handl J, Richard J. Worldwide occurrence of mycotoxins in commodities, feeds and feed ingredients. Animal Feed Science and Technology. 2007; **137**(3):265-282. ISSN: 0377-8401

[12] Mahmood S, Younus M, Aslam A, Anjum AA. Toxicological effects of aflatoxin B_1 on growth performance, humoral immune response and blood profile of japanese quail. Journal of Animal and Plant Sciences. 2017;**27**(3):833-840. ISSN: 1018-7081

[13] Placinta CM, D'Mello JPF, Macdonald AMC. A review of worldwide contamination of cereal grains and animal feed with Fusarium mycotoxins. Animal Feed Science and Technology. 1999;**78**:21-37

[14] Frisvad JC, Thrane U, Samson RA. Mycotoxin producers. In: Dijksterhuis J, Samson RA, editors. Food Mycology. A Multifaceted Approach to Fungi and Food. Boca Raton: CRC Press; 2007. pp. 135-159

[15] Casteel SW, Rottinghouse GE. Mycotoxicoses. Encyclopedia of Microbiology. 2000;**3**:337-348

[16] Ellis WO, Smith JP, Simpson BK, Oldham JH. Aflatoxins in food: Occurrence, biosynthesis effects on organisms, detection, and methods of control. Critical Reviews in Food Science and Nutrition. 1991;**30**:403-439

[17] Manal MZ, El-Midany SA, Shaheen HM, Rizzi L. Mycotoxins in animals: Occurrence, effects, prevention and management. Journal of Toxicology and Environmental Health Sciences. 2012;**4**(1):13-28. ISSN: 2006-9820. DOI: 10.5897/JTEHS11.072

[18] Filazi A, Begum YD, Ozgur K, Ufuk TS. Poultry science. Chapter: 4. In: Mycotoxins in Poultry. Rijeka: Intech; 2017. DOI: 10.5772/66302

[19] Maurice OM. Risk assessment for afatoxins in foodstuffs. International Biodeterioration and Biodegradation. 2002;**50**:137-142

[20] Pitt JI, Hocking AD. Fungi and Food Spoilage. Vol. 82. New South Wales, Australia: Blackie Academic & Professional; 1997

[21] Wilson DM, Payne GA. Factors Affecting Aspergillus fla6usgroup Infection and Aflatoxin Contamination of Crops. San Diego: Academic Press; 1994

[22] Ghahri H, Habibian R, Fam MA. Effect of sodium bentonites, mannan oligosaccharide and humate on performance and serum biochemical parameters during aflatoxicosis in broiler chickens. Global Veterinaria. 2010;**5**(2):129-134

[23] Williams JH, Phillips TD, Jolly PE, Stiles JK, Jolly CM, Aggarwal D. Human aflatoxicosis in developing countries: A review of toxicology, exposure, potential health consequences, and interventions. The American Journal of Clinical Nutrition. 2004;**80**(5):1106-1122

[24] Verma RJ. Aflatoxin cause DNA damage. International Journal of Human Genetics. 2004; **4**(4):231-236. ISSN: 0972-3757

[25] Elzupir AO, Younis YMH, Fadul MH, Elhussein AM. Determination of Aflatoxins in animal feed in Khartoum state, Sudan. Journal of Animal and Veterinary Advances. 2009;**8**(5):1000-1003. ISSN: 1680-5593

[26] Shareef AM. Molds and mycotoxins in poultry feeds from farms of potential mycotoxicosis. Iraqi Journal of Veterinary Sciences. 2010;**24**(1):17-25

[27] Anjum MA, Sahota WW, Akram M, Ali I. Prevalence of mycotoxins in poultry feeds and feed ingredients in Punjab (Pakistan). Journal of Animal and Plant Sciences. 2011;**21**(2): 117-120

[28] Bokhari FM. Aflatoxin production by Aspergillus flavus, isolated from differnt foodstuffs commonly used in Jeddah region, Saudi Arabia. Pakistan Journal of Biological Sciences. 2002;**5**(1):69-74

[29] Luttfullah G, Hussain A. Studies on contamination level of aflatoxins in some dried fruits and nuts of Pakistan. Food Control. 2011;**22**(3):426-429. ISSN. 0956-7135. DOI. 10.1016/j. food cont.2010.09.015

[30] Lutfullah G, Arshad H. Studies on contamination level of aflatoxins in some cereals and beans of Pakistan. Food Control. 2012;**23**:32-36

[31] Shah HU, Thomas JS, Sahib A, Khanzadi FK, Sajida P. Mould incidence and mycotoxin contamination in maize kernels from Swat Valley, north west Frontier Province of Pakistan. Food and Chemical Toxicology. 2010;**48**:1111-1116

[32] Borutova R, Aragon YA, Nährer K, Berthiller F. Co-occurrence and statistical correlations between mycotoxins in feedstuffs collected in the Asia–Oceania in 2010. Animal Feed Science and Technology. 2012;**178**(3–4):190-197. ISSN: 0377-8401. DOI: 10.1016/j.anifeedsci. 2012.09.015 URL: http://www.sciencedirect.com/science/article/pii/S0377840112003458

[33] Mardani M, Rezapour S, Rezapour P. Survey of aflatoxins in Kashkineh: A traditional Iranian food. Iranian Journal of Microbiology. 2011;**3**(3):147-151

[34] Brase S, Encinas A, Keck J, Nising CF. Chemistry and biology of mycotoxins and related fungal metabolites. Chemical Reviews. 2009;**109**:3903-4399

[35] IARC. Some traditional herbal medicines, some mycotoxins, naphthalene and styrene. IARC Monographs on the Evaluation of Carcinogenic Risks to Humans. 2002;**82**:1-556. PMID:12687954

[36] Azizollah K, Abdoullah H, Sudabeh M. Effect of yeast glucomannan on performance of broiler chicken. International Journal of Agriculture and Biology. 2009;**11**(1):49-53. ISSN: 1814-9596. DOI: 10.08-176/RNP/2009/11-1-49-53. URL: http://www.fspublishers.org

[37] Bhatnagar D, Rajesekaran K, Payne GA, Brown RI, Ye J, Cleveland TE. The 'omics' tools: Genomics, proteomics, metabolomics and their potential for solving the aflatoxin contamination problem. World Mycotoxin Journal. 2008;**1**:1-10

[38] Bintvihok A. Controlling aflatoxin danger to duck and duck meat. World's Poultry Science Journal. 2011;**17**:18-20

[39] Bianchi MD, Oliveira CAF, Al-Buquirque R, Guerra JL, Correa B. Effects of prolonged oral administration of aflatoxin B_1 and fumonisin in broiler chickens. Poultry Science. 2005;**84**:1835-1840

[40] Weidenborner M. Encyclopedia of Food Mycotoxins. New York, London: Spronger Publisher Berlin; 2001

[41] Kim HH, Velmurugu R, Xiuhua L, Ganesharanee R, Wayne LB. Apparent ileal digestibility of amino acids in feed ingredients determined with broilers and layers. Journal of the Science of Food and Agriculture. 2007;**87**:47-53

[42] Richard JL. Some major mycotoxins and their mycotoxicoses—An overview. International Journal of Food Microbiology. 2007;**119**:3-10

[43] Wayne LB. Mycotoxin contamination of the feed supply chain: Implications for animal productivity and feed security. Animal Feed Science and Technology. 2012;**173**(1–2):134-158. ISSN: 0377-8401. DOI: 10.1016/j.anifeedsci.2011.12.014. URL: http://www.sciencedirect.com/science/article /pii/S0377840111005037

[44] Yu J-H, Keller N. Regulation of secondary metabolism in filamentous fungi. Annual Review of Phytopathology. 2005;**43**:437-458. ISSN: 0066-4286

[45] Wu F, Miller JD, Casman EA. The economic impact of Bt corn resulting from mycotoxin reduction. Journal of Toxicology - Toxin Reviews. 2004;**23**:397-424

[46] Munkvold GP. Cultural and genetic approaches to managing mycotoxins in maize. Annual Review of Phytopathology. 2003;**41**:99-116

[47] Denli M, Blandon JC, Guynot ME, Salado S, Perez JF. Effects of dietary AflaDetox on performance, serum biochemistry, histopathological changes, and aflatoxin residues in broilers exposed to aflatoxin B_1. Poultry Science. 2009;**88**:1444-1451

[48] Quist CF, Bounous DI, Kilburn JV, Nettles VF, Wyatt RD. The effects of dietary aflatoxin on wild Turkey poults. Journal of Wildlife Diseases. 2000;**36**(3):436-444

[49] Patterson DSP. Metabolism as a factor in determining the toxic action of the aflatoxins in different animal species. Food and Cosmetics Toxicology. 1973;**11**:287-294

[50] Chen X, Horn N, Cotter PF, Applegate TJ. Growth, serum biochemistry, complement activity, and liver gene expression responses of Pekin ducklings to graded levels of cultured aflatoxin B_1. Poultry Science. 2014;**93**:2028-2036. DOI: 10.3382/ps.2014-03904

[51] Suksombat W, Suksombat P, Mirttanaphari R. Effect of commercial or bovine yeasts on the performance and blood variables of broiler chickens intoxicated with Aflatoxins. World Academy of Science, Engineering and Technology. 2011;**58**:664-668

[52] Morrison DM, David RL, Lambert FBC, Coretta ANS. A limited survey of aflatoxins in poultry feed and feed ingredients in Guyana. Journal of Veterinary Science. 2017;**60**(4):1-7. DOI: 10.3390/vetsci4040060

[53] Santin E, Paulillo AC, Nakagui LSO, Alessi AC, Maiorka A. Evaluation of yeast cell wall on the performance of broiler fed diets with or without mycototoxins. Brazilian Journal of Poultry Science. 2006;**8**(4):221-225. ISSN: 1516-635X (Print), 1806-9061 (online). DOI: 10.1590/S1516-635X2006000400004

[54] Stewart BW, Kleihues P. World Cancer Report. Geneva; 2003

[55] Zaghini A, Martelli G, Roncada P, Simioli M, Rizzi L. Mannan-oligosaccharides and aflatoxin B_1 in feed for laying hens: Effects on egg quality, afltxonins B_1 and M_1 residues in eggs, and aflatoxin B_1 levels in liver. Poultry Science. 2005;**84**:825-832. ISSN: 0032-5791. DOI: 10.1093/ps/84.6.825

[56] Gallagher EP, Wienkers LC, Stapleton PL, Kunze KL, Eaton DL. Role of human microsomal & human complementary DNA-expressed cytochromes P4501A2 and P4503A4 in the bioactivation of aflatoxin B_1. Cancer Research. 1994;**54**:101-108

[57] Lillehoj EB, Cleveland TE, Bhatnagar D. Mycotoxins in Feedstuffs: Production in Novel Substrates. Florida, Boca Raton: CRC Press; 1991. p. 399

[58] Gan LS, Skipper PL, Peng XC, Groopman JD, Chen JS, Wogan GN, et al. Serum albumin adducts in the molecular epidemiology of aflatoxin carcinogenesis: Correlation with aflatoxin B_1 intake and urinary excretion of aflatoxin M_1. Carcinogenesis. 1988;**9**:1323-1325

[59] Li JJ, Suo D, Su XO. Binding capacity for aflatoxin B_1 by different adsorbents. Agricultural Sciences in China. 2010;**9**(3):449-456. ISSN: 1671-2927. DOI: 10.1016/S1671-2927(09)60116-4

[60] Gopalakrishnan S, Harris TM, Stone MP. International of aflatoxin B_1 in two oligodeoxynucleotide adducts: Comparative 1H NMR analysis of d (ATCAFBGAT). d(ATCGAT) and d(ATFBGCAT)$_2$. The Biochemist. 1990;**29**:10438-10448

[61] Kobertz WR, Wang D, Wogan GN, Essigmann JM. An intercalation inhibitor alerting the target selectivity of DNA damagingagents; synthesis of site-specific aflatoxin B_1 adducts in a p53 mutational hotspot. Proceedings of the National Academy of Sciences of the United States of America. 1997;**94**:9579-9584

[62] Groopman JD, Donahue PR, Zhu J, Chen J, Wogan GN. Aflatoxin metabolism in humans: Detection of metabolites and nucleic acid adducts in urine by affinity chromatography. Proceedings of the National Academy of Sciences of the United States of America. 1985; **82**:6492-6496. ISSN: 0027-8424

[63] Haschek WM, Voss KA, Beasley VR. Selected Mycotoxins Affecting Animal and Human Health. 2nd ed. Vol. 1. New York: Academic Press; 2002. pp. 645-699

[64] Surai PF. Natural antioxidants and mycotoxins. In: Natural Antioxidants in Avian Nutrition and Reproduction. UK: Nottingham University Press; 2002. pp. 455-489

[65] Wild CP, Turner PC. Exposure biomarkers in chemoprevention studies of liver cancer. I. A.R.C. 2001;**154**:215-222

[66] Montesano R, Hainaut P, Wild CP. Hepatocellular carcinoma: From gene to public health. Journal of the National Cancer Institute. 1997;**89**:1844-1851

[67] Puisieux A, Lim S, Groopman J, Ozturk M. Selective targeting of p53 gene mutational hotspots in human cancers by etiologically defined carcinogen. Cancer Research. 1991; **51**:6158-6189

[68] Hendrickse RG. Clinical implications of food contaminated by aflatoxins. Annals of the Academy of Medicine, Singapore. 1991;**20**:84-90

[69] Fernandez A, Verde MT, Gascon M, Ramos J, Gomez J, Luco DF, et al. Variations of clinical biochemical parameters of laying hens and broiler chickens fed aflatoxin containing feed. Avian Pathology. 1994;**23**:37-47

[70] Donmez N, Keskin E. The effect of aflatoxin and glucomannan on some antioxidants and biochemical parameters in rabbits. Acta Veterinaria. 2008;**58**(4):307-313. DOI: 10.2298/AVB0804307D

[71] Hussain Z, Khan MZ, Khan A, Javed I, Saleemi MK, Mahmood S, et al. Residues of aflatoxin B_1 in broiler meat: Effect of age and dietary aflatoxin B_1 levels. Food and Chemical Toxicology. 2010;**48**(12):3304-3307. ISSN: 0278-6915. DOI: 10.1016/j.fct.2010.08.016. URL: http://www.sciencedirect.com/science/article/pii/S0278691510005260

[72] Fowler J, Wei L, Christopher B. Effects of a calcium bentonite clay in diets containing aflatoxin when measuring liver residues of aflatoxin B_1 in starter broiler chicks. Toxins. 2015;**7**(9):3455-3464. DOI: 10.3390/toxins7093455

[73] Lakkawar AW, Narayanaswamy HD, Satyanarayana ML. Study on efficacy of diatomaceous earth to ameliorate aflatoxin - induced pathomorphological changes in lymphoid organs of broiler chicken. Veterinária. 2017;**66**(3):111-117

[74] Richard JL, Pier AC, Cysewski SJ, Graham CK. Effect of aflatoxin and aspergillosis on Turkey poults. 1973;**17**(1):111-121. ISSN: 00052086. DOI: 10.2307/1588926. URL: http://www.jstor.org/stable/1588926

[75] Bondy G, Pestka JJ. Immunomodulation by fungal toxins. Journal of Toxicology & Environmental Health Part B: Critical Reviews. 2000;**3**:109-143. ISSN: 1093-7404. DOI: 10.1080/109374000281113

[76] Huff WE, Kubena LF, Harvey RB, Corrier DE, Mollenhauer HH. Progression of aflatoxicosis in broiler chickens. Poultry Science. 1986;**65**:1891-1899

[77] Reddy DVR, Thirumala-Devi K, Reddy SV, Waliyar F, Mayo MA, Devi KR, et al. Estimation of Aflatoxin levels in selected foods and feeds in India. In: International Workshop.

France: CIRAD-FAO; 2000. pp. 11-13. URL: http://www.researchgate.net/publication/237814423

[78] Richard JL, Payne GA, Desjardins AE, Maragos C, Norred WP, Pestka JJ. Mycotoxins: Risks in plant, animal and human systems. CAST Task Force Report. 2003;**139**:101-103

[79] Pier C. Major biological consequences of aflatoxicosis in animal production. Journal of Animal Science. 1992;**70**:3964-3967

[80] Oswald IP, Martin DE, Bouhet S, Pinton P, Taranu I, Accensi F. Immunotoxiological risk of mycotoxins for domestic animals. Food Additives and Contaminants. 2005;**22**(4):354-360. ISSN: 0265-203X. DOI: 10.1080/02652030500058320

[81] Meissonnier GM, Pinton P, Laffitte J, Cossalter A-M, Gong YY, Wild CP, et al. Immunotoxicity of aflatoxin B_1: Impairment of cell-mediated response to vaccine antigen and modulation of cytokine expression. Toxicology and Applied Pharmacology. 2008;**231**(2):142-149. ISSN: 0041-008X. DOI: 10.1016/j.taap.2008.04.004

[82] Chang C-F, Hamilton PB. Refractory phagocytosis by chicken thrombocytes during aflatoxicosis. Poultry Science. 1979;**58**:559-561. ISSN: 0032-5791. DOI: 10.3382/ps.0580559

[83] Vincelli P, Parker G, McNeill S, Smith RA, Woloshuk C, Coffey R, Overhults DG. Aflatoxins in Corn. ID-59. USA: College of Agriculture, University of Kentucky; 1995. URL: http://www.ca.uky.edu/agc/pubs/id/id59/id59.pdf

[84] Frank TJ, Winston MH, Pat BH. Correlation of aflatoxin contaminated with zinc content of chicken feed. Applied and Environmental Microbiology. 1984;**47**(3):478-480. ISSN: 0099-2240

[85] Rawal S, Ji EK, Roger C. Aflatoxin B_1in poultry: Toxicology, metabolism and prevention. Research in Veterinary Science. 2010;**89**(3):325-331

[86] Diaz DE, Smith TK. Mycotoxins sequestering agents: Practical tools for neutralization of mycotoxins. In: The Mycotoxin Blue Book. England: Nottingham University Press; 2005. pp. 323-339. ISBN. 1904761194

[87] Rosa CA, Mizzo R, Magnoli C, Salvano M, Chiac SM, Ferrero S, et al. Evaluation of the efficacy of bentonite from the south of Argentina to ameliorate the toxic effects of aflatoxin in broilers. Poultry Science. 2001;**80**:139-144

[88] Kabak B. The fate of mycotoxins during thermal food processing. Journal of the Science of Food and Agriculture. 2009;**89**:549-554 . ISSN: 1097-0010. DOI: 10.1002/jsfa.3491

[89] Huwig A, Freimund S, Käppeli O, Dutler H. Mycotoxin detoxication of animal feed by different adsorbents. Toxicology Letters. 2001;**122**:179-188. ISSN: 0378-4274. DOI: 10.1016/S0378-4274(01)00360-5

[90] Jalili M, Jinap S, Son R. The effect of chemical treatment on reduction of aflatoxins and ochratoxin a in black and white pepper during washing. Food Additives and Contaminants. 2011;**28**(4):485-493. ISSN: 1944-0049. DOI: 10.1080/19440049.2010.551300

[91] Park DL, Price WD. Reduction of aflatoxin hazards using ammoniation. In: Rev Environ Contam Toxicol, Aflatoxin Reduction. Vol. 171. Springer-Verlag; 2001. pp. 139-175. ISBN. 0179-5953

[92] Edlayne G, Simone A, Felicio JD. Chemical and biological approaches for mycotoxin control: A review. Recent Patents on Food, Nutrition & Agriculture. 2009;**1**(2):155-161. ISSN: 2212-7984

[93] Kolossova A, Stroka J. Evaluation of the effect of mycotoxin binders in animal feed on the analytical performance of standardised methods for the determination of mycotoxins in feed. 2009;**29**(12):1959-1971. ISSN: 1944–0049 (print), 1944–0057 (online). DOI: 10.1080/19440049.2012.720035

[94] Phillips TD, Sarr AB, Clement BA, Kubena LF, Harvey RB. Prevention of aflatoxicosis in farm animals via selective chemiosorption of aflatoxin. In: Bray GA, Ryan DH, editors. Mycotoxins, Cancer and Health. Vol 1. Baton Rouge: Louisiana State University Press; 1991. pp. 223-237

[95] Schiedeler SE. Effects of various types of aluminosilicates and aflatoxin B_1 on aflatoxin toxicity, chick performance, and mineral status. Poultry Science. 1993;**72**(2):282-288. ISSN: 0032-5791. DOI: 10.3382/ps.0720282

[96] Mahesh BK, Devegowda G. Ability of aflatoxin binders to bind aflatoxin in contaminated poultry feeds- an *in vitro* study. In: XX World's Poultry Congress. Vol. 4. 1996. p. 296

[97] Magnoli AP, Tallone L, Rosa RCA, Dalcero AM, Chiacchiera SM, Sanchez RMT. Structural characteristic of commercial bentonites used as detoxifier of broiler feed contamination with aflatoxin. Applied Clay Science. 2008;**40**:63-71

[98] Daković A, Tomašević-Čanović M, Dondur D, Vujaković A, Radošević P. Kinetics of aflatoxin B_1 and G_2 adsorption on Ca-clinoptilolite. Journal of the Serbian Chemical Society. 2000;**65**(10):715-723. ISSN: 0352-5139

[99] Grant PG, Phillips TD. Isothermal adsorption of aflatoxin B_1 on HSCAS clay. Journal of Agricultural and Food Chemistry. 1998;**46**:599-605. ISSN: 0021-8561

[100] Ramos AJ, Hernández E, Plá-Delfina M, Merino M. Intestinal absorption of zearalenone and *in vitro* study of non- nutritive sorbent materials. International Journal of Pharmaceutics. 1996;**128**(1):129-137. ISSN: 0378-5173. DOI: 10.1016/0378-5173(95)04239-3

[101] Pasha TN, Mahmood A, Khattak FM, Jabbar MA, Khan AD. The effect of feed supplemented with different sodium bentonite treatments on broiler performance. Turkish Journal of Veterinary and Animal Sciences. 2008;**32**(4):245-248

[102] Safaeikatouli M, Jafariahangari Y, Baharlouei A. An evaluation on the effects of dietary kaolin and zeolite on broilers blood parameters, T4, TSH and growth hormones. Pakistan Journal of Nutrition. 2011;**10**:233-237

[103] Tomašević-Čanović M, Daković A, Marković V, Stojšić D. The effect of exchangeable cations in clinoptiololite and montmorillonite on the absorption of aflatoxin B_1. Journal of the Serbian Chemical Society. 2001;**66**(8):555-561

[104] Phillips TD, Lemke SL, Grant PG. Characterization of clay-based enterosorbents for the prevention of aflatoxicosis. Advances in Experimental Medicine and Biology, Mycotoxins and Food Safety. 2002;**504**:157-171. ISBN. 1461351669

[105] Eleroğlu H, Yalçın H, Yıldırım A. Dietary effects of ca-zeolite supplementation on some blood and tibial bone characteristics of broilers. South African Journal Of Animal Science. 2011;**41**(4):330. ISSN: 0375-1589 (print), 222-4062 (online)-319. DOI: 10.4314/sajas.v41i4.1

[106] Khanedar F, Vakili R, Zakizadeh S. Effects of two kinds of bentonite on the performance, blood biochemical parameters, carcass characteristics and tibia ash of broiler chicks. Global Veterinaria. 2012;**9**(6):720-725. ISSN: 1992-6197. DOI: 10.5829/idosi.gv.2012.9.6.61151

[107] Kececi T, Oguz H, Kurtoglu V, Demet O. Effects of polyvinyl polypyrolidone, synthetic zeolite and bentonite on serum biochemical and haematological characters of broiler chickens during aflatoxicosis. British Poultry Science. 1998;**39**:452-458. ISSN: 0007-1668. DOI: 10.1080/00071669889051

[108] Southern LL, Ward TL, Bidner TD, Hebert LG. Effects of sodium bentonite or hydrated sodium calcium aluminosilicate on growth performance and tibia mineral concentrations in broiler chicks fed nutrient deficient diets. Poultry Science. 1994;**73**(6):848-854. ISSN: 0032-5791. DOI: 10.3382/ps.0730848

[109] Chestnut AB, Anderson PD, Cochran MA, Fribourg HA, Twinn KD. Effect of hydrated sodium calcium aluminosilicate on fescue toxicosis and mineral absorption. Journal of Animal Science. 1992;**70**:2838-2846. ISSN: 0021-8812. DOI: /1992.7092838x

[110] Kramer K, Anke M, Glei M, Muller M. Effects of oral bentonite offer on macro and trace element incorporation of different parts of the body and the milk. In: Anke M, Meissner D, Mills CF, editors. Trace Elements in Man and Animals. Germany: Verlag Medica Touristik, Gersdorf; 1993. pp. 466-469

[111] Solís-Cruz B, Hernández-Patlán D, Beyssac E, Latorre JD, Hernandez-Velasco X, Merino-Guzman R, et al. Evaluation of chitosan and cellulosic polymers as binding adsorbent materials to prevent aflatoxin B_1, fumonisin B_1, ochratoxin, trichothecene, deoxynivalenol, and zearalenone mycotoxicoses through an in vitro gastrointestinal model for poultry. Polymer. 2017;**9**:529. DOI: 10.3390/polym9100529

[112] Shetty PH, Jespersen L. *Saccharomyces cerevisiae* and lactic acid bacteria as potential mycotoxin decontaminating agents. Trends in Food Science and Technology. 2006;**17**(2): 48-55. ISSN: 0924-2244. DOI: 10.1016/j.tifs.2005.10.004

[113] Turbic A, Ahokas JT, Haskard CA. Selective *in vitro* binding of dietary mutagens, individually or in combination, by lactic acid bacteria. Food Additives and Contaminants. 2002;**19**:144-152. ISSN: 0265-203X. DOI: 10.1080/02652030110070067

[114] van der Aa Kühle A, Skovgaard K, Jespersen L. *In vitro* screening of probiotic properties of *Saccharomyces cerevisiae* var. boulardii and food borne *Saccharomyces cerevisiae* strains. International Journal of Food Microbiology. 2004;**101**(1):29-40. ISSN: 0168-1605. DOI: 10.1016/j.ijfoodmicro.2004.10.039

[115] Ouwehand AC, Niemi P, Salminen SJ. The normal faecal microflora does not affect the adhesion of probiotic bacteria *in vitro*. FEMS Microbiology Letters. 1999;**177**(1):35-38. ISSN: 0378-1097. DOI: 10.1111/j.1574-6968.1999.tb13710.x

[116] Coallier-Ascah J, Idziak ES. Interaction between *Streptococcus lactis* and *Aspergillus flavus* on production of aflatoxin. Applied and Environmental Microbiology. 1985;**49**:163-167. ISSN: 0099-2240

[117] Thyagaraja N, Hosono A. Binding properties of lactic acid bacteria from 'idly' towards food-borne mutagens. Food and Chemical Toxicology. 1994;**32**(9):805-809. ISSN: 0278-6915. DOI: 10.1016/0278-6915(94)90156-2

[118] Haskard CA, El-Nezami HS, Peltonen KD, Salminen S, Ahokas JT. Sequestration of aflatoxin B_1 by probiotic strains: Binding capacity and localization. Revista de Medicina Veterinaria. 1998;**149**:571. ISSN: 0035-1555

[119] Haskard C, Binnion C, Ahokas J. Factors affecting the sequestration of aflatoxin by *Lactobacillus rhamnosusstrain GG*. Chemico-Biological Interactions. 2000;**128**:39-49. ISSN: 0009-2797. DOI: 10.1016/S0009-2797(00)00186-1

[120] Lahtinen SJ, Haskard CA, Ouwehandz AC, Salminenz SJ, Ahokasy JT. Binding of aflatoxin B_1 to cell wall components of *Lactobacillus rhamnosus* strain GG. Food Additives and Contaminants. 2004;**21**(2):158-164. ISSN: 0265-203X. DOI: 10.1080/02652030310001639521

[121] Lewis SJ, Freedman AR. Review article: The use of biotherapeutic agents in the prevention and treatment of gastrointestinal disease. Alimentary Pharmacology & Therapeutics. 1998;**12**(9):807-822. ISSN: 1365-2036

[122] Kusumaningtyas E, Widiastuti R, Maryam R. Reduction of aflatoxin B_1 in chicken using *Saccharomyces cerevisiae, Rhizopus* and their combination. Mycopathologia. 2006;**162**(4): 307-311. ISSN: 0301-486X. DOI: 10.1007/s11046-006-0047-4

[123] Celyk K, Denly M, Savas T. Reduction of toxic effects of aflatoxin B_1 by using baker yeast (*Saccharomyces cerevisiae*) in growing broiler chicks diets. Revista Brasileira de Zootecnia. 2003;**32**(3):615-619. DOI: 10.1590/S1516-35982003000300013

[124] Šari L, Marija MŠ, Marijana BS, Dragana VP, Abarkapa IS. Effect of the baker's yeast on the production of aflatoxin B_1 by *Aspergillus flavus*. Food Process Quality Safety. 2008; **35**(4):165-168. ISSN: 1821-0554

[125] Yiannikouris A, Francois J, Poughon L, Dussap CG, Jeminet G, Bertin G. Influence of pH on complexing of model b-D-glucans with zearalenone. Journal of Food Protection. 2004;**67**: 2741-2746

[126] Devegowda G, Arvind BIR, Morton MG. *Saccharomyces Cerevisiae* and mannan Ooligosaccharides to counteract aflatoxicosis in broilers. In: Austr Poult Sci Symp; 1996. pp. 103-106

[127] Murthy TNK, Devegowda G. Efficacy of modified glucomannan (Mycosorb) to adsorb aflatoxin B1 in gut conditions of broiler chickens. In: XXII World's Poultry Congress, Istanbul, Turkey; 2004

Chapter 8

Control of Aflatoxicosis in Poultry Using Probiotics and Polymers

Bruno Solis-Cruz, Daniel Hernandez-Patlan,
Billy M. Hargis and Guillermo Tellez

Additional information is available at the end of the chapter

http://dx.doi.org/10.5772/intechopen.76371

Abstract

An important approach to prevent aflatoxicosis in poultry is the addition of non-nutritional adsorbents in the diet to bind aflatoxin B1 (AFB1) in the gastrointestinal tract. These adsorbents are large molecular weight compounds that are able to bind the mycotoxin, forming a stable complex adsorbent-mycotoxin, which can pass through the gastrointestinal tract. In this chapter, we evaluate the use of polymers and probiotics to reduce AFB1 toxic effects in poultry. Our results on the efficacy of polymers and probiotics in sequestering mycotoxins are highly promising, although this field is still in its infancy and further research is needed. Furthermore, *in vivo* studies are needed to confirm the effectiveness of these materials against AFB1 toxic effects, since results in the past have indicated that there is great variability in the efficacy of adsorbing materials *in vivo*, even though the compounds may show potential adsorption capacity of the mycotoxin *in vitro*.

Keywords: aflatoxins, chickens, polymers, adsorption, probiotics

1. Introduction

Mycotoxins are low molecular weight compounds produced as secondary metabolites by filamentous fungi contaminating crops in the field or warehouses when environmental conditions of temperature and humidity are adequate. These metabolites have no biochemical relevance to fungal growth or development, and they constitute a chemically and toxicologically heterogeneous group, which are together only because they can cause diseases, including death, to human beings and other animals even at low concentrations [1].

Currently, more than 400 different mycotoxins are known, but only six are currently considered to be of worldwide importance, and aflatoxins are the most toxigenic and investigated mycotoxins worldwide because their natural occurrence can cause serious economic losses and health problems [2, 3]. In terms of toxicity and occurrence, aflatoxin B1 (AFB1) is the most important mycotoxin due to its hepatotoxic and hepatocarcinogenic effects, which can result in immunosuppression, anorexia with reduced growth rate, decreased egg production, reduced reproductivity, poor feed utilization, anemia, hemorrhage, and increased mortality [4, 5]. Furthermore, intoxication with AFB1 has been linked to other severe effects such as teratogenesis, carcinogenesis, and mutagenesis [6].

Due to the severe and harmful effects of AFB1, many methods to reduce its toxic effects have been proposed. The first and best attempt to prevent the effects of AFB1 is to minimize its production through good agricultural practices (GAP), including cultivating practices in fields as well as harvest, transport, and storage conditions [7, 8], all these steps are under GAP. However, since prevention is not always possible, decontaminating and/or detoxifying methods have been gaining attention as an alternative to reducing AFB1 contamination of feed and grains. Methods of detoxification can be physical, chemical, or biological treatments of contaminated feed or grains, and they can be as simple as the physical separation through screening, classification, and selection of damaged grains or as complex as gamma irradiation or chemical methods using ammonia, ozone, hydrogen peroxide, or some acids and alkalis [9–14]. Nevertheless, many of these methods to detoxify aflatoxin-contaminated feed are not currently available because they cannot be applied on a large scale and in a cost-effective manner or because many of them are impractical, ineffective, or potentially unsafe.

Another approach to prevent aflatoxicosis in animals is the addition of adsorbents in the diet for binding aflatoxin in the gastrointestinal tract so that these compounds impede its adsorption in the intestine [15]. Adsorbents have been recurrently used because of their economic feasibility and suitability for nutritional perspective [16]. Many studies have demonstrated that aluminosilicates, mainly zeolites, hydrated sodium calcium aluminosilicate (HSCAS), and aluminosilicate-containing clays, can effectively reduce aflatoxins toxicity to animals; being these inorganic materials, the most thoroughly studied adsorbents [17–21]. Alternatively, both carbon-based organic polymers and synthetic polymers have been tested, and some of them are currently on the market [17, 22]. Even though the cost of these polymers could be the limiting factor for practical applications, their use can help to solve the problems related with the use of aluminosilicates and clay adsorbents, such as binding preferly just to aflatoxins, the possibility to adsorb important micronutrients, and the risk of natural clays to be contaminated with dioxins [7, 23]. Nowadays, there are some highly promising research on the effectiveness of synthetic and organic polymers in adsorbing aflatoxins, although this field is still under developing and it needs more *in vitro* and *in vivo* research [24].

On the other hand, biological methods to prevent aflatoxicosis have also been evaluated showing promising results [25–28]. Many microorganisms, including bacteria, yeasts, molds, actinomycetes, and algae,. have been tested for their ability in the control of aflatoxin contamination, mainly through adsorption and degradation [29, 30]. Among the bacteria tested, probiotics have been identified as a good option to reduce the availability of aflatoxins *in vitro*. Additionally, probiotic bacteria have shown numerous beneficial health effects, which make them even more suitable additives to food and feed [25, 31–33].

2. Biological importance of AFB1 in poultry

Poultry species are probably the most sensitive food-producing animals to AFB1 toxic effects, and small amounts of it severely damage animal health and the profitability of the productive system, which results in substantial annual economic losses to producers [6, 34–39].

However, there are also differences in terms of susceptibility to AFB1 among poultry species, which could be due to differences in hepatic metabolism of AFB1 in these species. According to comparative toxicological studies, ducklings and turkey poults are the most sensitive species to AFB1, followed by goslings and young pheasants with intermediate sensitivity, and finally, the chicks showed to have relative resistance to AFB1 injury [40]. Toxicity and carcinogenicity of AFB1 occur after its bioactivation by the cytochrome P450 (CYP450) mixed function oxidase system, resulting in a highly reactive AFB1 8,9-epoxide (AFBO), which forms covalent adducts with cellular macromolecules such as DNA, RNA, protein constituents, and some enzymes [41–44]. Since metabolic activation of AFB1 to AFBO by CYP450 is especially efficient in poultry species [45], they are extreme sensitivity to the toxic effects of AFB1. Another possible reason which may also explain the differences in susceptibility of poultry species is the variation in phase II biotransformation enzymes, such as glutathione S-transferase (GST), that catalyze a conjugation reaction of AFBO with endogenous glutathione (GSH). Although avian species are highly efficient in producing AFBO, they are not able to conjugate it effectively with GSH, which indicates that they have low GST activity [46, 47].

The most noticeable effect of AFB1 on poultry is the impair of all important productive parameters, including body weight gain, feed intake, feed conversion efficiency, pigmentation, processing yield, egg production, male and female reproductive performance, and an increased mortality [35, 48, 49]. These alterations in the productive parameters are the result of the physiological effects of AFB1 consumption, of which liver damage is the most notorious, characterized by its enlargement, pale yellow coloration, petechial hemorrhages and hematomas on the surface, usually accompanied with proliferation of biliary ducts and depletion of lymphoid organs [50–52]. However, for poultry industry AFB1 contamination and consumption are important because of its ability to decrease resistance to common infectious diseases, including parasitic, bacterial, and viral infections, due to depression of the humoral and cellular immune responses [53–57].

3. Microbiological control of AFB1

To date, many physical and chemical methods have been used to detoxify AFB1; however, only a few of these methods are in practical use, probably due to difficulties in complying with the FAO requirements: reduction of AFB1 without residual toxicity, guarantee of nutritional values, and no modification of food or feed properties [58, 59]. Since cost-effective methods to detoxify mycotoxin-contaminated grains and foods are urgently needed to minimize potential losses to the farmer and toxicological hazards to the consumer [60], finding of new and suitable methods for AFB1 decontamination has become a primary need.

In this sense, microbiological control approach has taken strength in the field of research to control AFB1. Researchers have focused on biological treatments for detoxification mainly through two mechanisms: adsorption and degradation, both of which can be achieved by biological systems such as bacteria, yeasts, molds, actinomycetes, and algae [61].

Biological adsorption can occur either by attaching the AFB1 to the cell wall components of the microorganisms or by active internalization and accumulation. Also, dead microorganisms can absorb AFB1, and this phenomenon can be exploited in the creation of biofilters for fluid decontamination or probiotics to bind and remove the AFB1 from the intestine [62]. However, biological adsorption mechanism is naturally reversible, and AFB1 may be easily released, so that it is necessary to search for novel approaches to overcome these drawbacks, as for example the combination of mineral and biological adsorbents to improve their effectiveness [63].

On the other hand, microbiological biodegradation is performed by either extracellular or intracellular enzymes, so the degradation is generally permanent and irreversible which can alter, reduce, or completely eradicate AFB1 toxicity [30]. Nevertheless, modification of AFB1 structure can result in other molecules, such as aflatoxicol (AFL), also with potential toxic effects [64]. Thus, further knowledge is needed on the identification, quantity, and toxicity of degradation metabolites prior to the potential applications of biological treatments [59].

Microbiological control seems to be becoming one of the most promising approaches for AFB1 control; since the last four decades, the use of microorganisms is one of the well-known strategies for the management of AFB1 in foods and feeds. These methods of bioadsorption and biodegradation are being actively studied and can be a highly promising choice because they are efficient, specific, and environmentally friendly [65–68].

4. Use of probiotics to prevent AFB1 toxic effects in poultry

Microbiological control of AFB1 is still considered as a promising area in research; so recently, these methods have attracted researcher's attention due to their easy usage and affordable processes [69]. However, since the use of microorganisms is expected to be safe both for animal health and for the production of innocuous livestock products, there are still many microorganisms that cannot be directly employed in the food or feed directly. In the last decades, research to find microorganisms for AFB1 control has focused on testing, screening, and choosing those strains that have demonstrated their effectiveness not only to reduce or even suppress AFB1 toxicity but also to be Generally Regarded as Safe (GRAS) [70, 71].

There are several microorganisms that have been shown to be effective in preventing and controlling the toxic effects of AFB1; among them, probiotic bacterial strains are some of the most studied, due largely to their GRAS character and because they have shown to have several potential applications against AFB1 both *in vitro* and *in vivo* [72–75]. Probiotics are living microorganisms that when administered in adequate amounts confer a health benefit to the host directly or indirectly through the maintenance of the microbial balance in their digestive tract [65, 76]. Several bacterial genera have been used as probiotics in livestock, including many species of *Bacillus, Bifidobacterium, Enterococcus, E. coli, Lactobacillus, Lactococcus,* and *Streptococcus,* although some species of molds and yeasts, such as *Aspergillus, Candida,* and *Saccharomyces,* have also been used [77, 78].

In poultry industry, probiotics have been reported to have a beneficial effect on performance, modulation of intestinal microflora and pathogen inhibition, intestinal histological changes, immunomodulation, certain hematobiochemical parameters, improving sensory characteristics of dressed meat, and promoting microbiological meat quality [79, 80]. In addition, probiotic bacteria may possess antimutagenic and anticarcinogenic activity. The mechanisms of these activities remain unclear; however, alteration of fecal bacterial enzyme activities associated with conversion of promutagens and procarcinogens to ultimate carcinogens and binding of dietary mutagens and carcinogens has been proposed [81].

Three possible mechanisms have been proposed by which probiotics can counteract the toxic effects of AFB1: (1) competing with aflatoxigenic mold strains for space, occupying the same ecological niche or using nutrients, and thus reducing AFB1 biosynthesis; (2) encouraging AFB1 metabolic degradation by enzymes, or (3) impeding its intestinal absorption by AFB1 binding onto the cell walls of the probiotics strains.

It has been suggested by *in vitro* studies that probiotics can inhibit AFB1 production through releasing metabolites to the media, such as organic acids, bacteriocins, and even hydrogen peroxide, which may interfere with AFB1 biosynthesis [82, 83]. Other alternative could be the reduction or inhibition in the growth of aflatoxigenic mold strains caused by a decrease in pH of the media and/or a nutrient competition of the culture media, which could also have contributed to the removal of AFB1 [84–87]. In **Figure 1**, it is shown how some probiotics from the lactobacilli strains can decrease both AFB1 production and the growth rate of an aflatoxigenic mold strain.

Although several bacterial strains have been used as biocompetitive agents of aflatoxigenic mold strains, some of them become inactive under extreme conditions of humidity and temperature, so that not all probiotic strains are ideal for this application. In this sense, studies on the prevention of AFB1 contamination using highly competitive non-toxigenic strains of *A. parasiticus* and *A. flavus* have shown certain advantages, which implies that these mold strains may be potentially useful as agents directed at competitively excluding toxigenic strains [88].

The other mechanism that the probiotics have to counteract the toxic effects of AFB1 is through its metabolic degradation or biodegradation, which can be defined as the degradation or enzymatic transformation of the mycotoxin to less or non-toxic compounds. Biodegradation using microorganisms or their enzymes is one of the most studied strategies for AFB1 management; this method has been actively studied and can be a highly promising choice, since it is efficient, specific, and environmentally friendly to reduce or eliminate the possible contaminations of

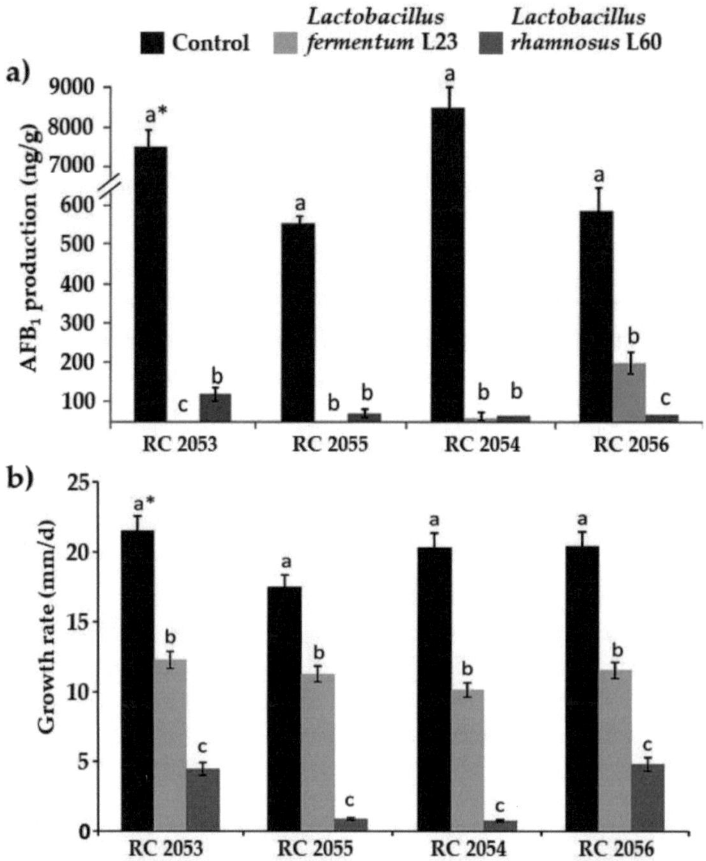

Figure 1. Effect of lactobacilli strains on: (a) the production of AFB1 and (b) the rate growth by *Aspergillus* section *Flavi*. Mean values based on quadruplicate data. * Mean with a letter in common is not significantly different according to Tukey's test ($p < 0.05$) (modified from [83]).

AFB1 under mild conditions, without using harmful chemicals and without significant impairment of the nutritive value or palatability of the detoxified food or feed [68].

Studies on microbial degradation of AFB1 involve the use of microbial catabolic pathways, which act on one of the two key sites influencing its toxicity and potency, shown in **Figure 2**. The first site is the double bond in position 1,2 of the furofuran ring [41], and the second reactive group is the lactone ring in the coumarin moiety [89]. AFB1 is usually detoxified to a less toxic compound by opening the lactone ring, altering the coumarin structure, but it can also occur by removing the double bond from furan ring when there is a scission on it [2, 90, 91]. It is known that opening the lactone ring abolishes or decreases the fluorescence spectrum of AFB1; however, the cleavage of the furofuran ring does not change its fluorescence properties [92].

For AFB1 metabolic degradation, several microbial isolates have been studied and reported with different levels of degradation capacities, including bacteria and fungi strains [94–101];

http://dx.doi.org/10.5772/intechopen.76371

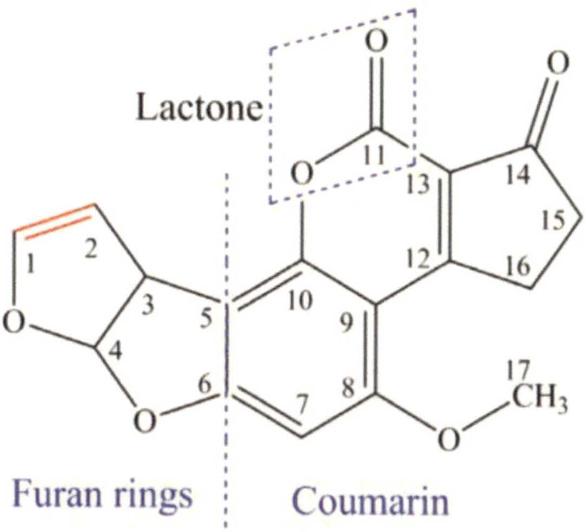

Figure 2. Chemical molecular structure of AFB1, showing the two key sites responsible of its toxicity (taken from [93]).

however, for the fungi species, limitations such as long degradation time, non-adaptability to typical food fermentations, and culture pigmentation reduced their potential application in AFB1 detoxification [97], besides the use of fungi species is not economical because of the extraction process and lengthy incubation time [102]. Moreover, some of these fungi strains with degradation potential may also produce AFB1 under varying conditions [103].

One of the first studies in this area was carried out in the 1960s, when it was evaluated the ability of about 1000 types of microorganisms to degrade aflatoxins [61]. Since then, many other studies have been done with several bacterial genera and strains; being the lactic acid bacteria (LAB), the most studied to detoxify AFB1; nevertheless, the ability of LABs to detoxify AFB1 has been attributed to their strong affinity and capacity to adsorb the toxin rather than for their degradation abilities [75, 81, 104–106].

AFB1 degrading activity has been found in other bacteria genera, such as *Mycobacterium fluoranthenivoran*, *Nocardia corynebacterioides* (formerly *Flavobacterium aurantiacum*), *Rhodococcus erythropolis*, *Stenotrophomonas maltophilia*, *Pseudomonas*, as well as *Bacillus licheniformis* and *B. subtilis* [70, 71, 97, 107–110], which have demonstrated that their biodegradation activity is from enzymatic nature. For example, *B. subtilis* JSW-1, a bacterium isolated from soil samples, is able to degrade almost 70% of AFB1 within 72 h, as shown in **Figure 3**, and its degradation activity was likely due to the extracellular enzymes [26]. In other study, biological degradation of AFB1 by *Rhodococcus erythropolis* was evaluated in liquid cultures, in which dramatic reduction of AFB1 was observed after 48 and 72 h of incubation with just 17 and 3–6% of residual AFB1, respectively [97]. The ability to effectively biotransform AFB1 by *Myxococcus fulvus* has also been demonstrated. This bacterial isolate from deer feces was able to biotransform AFB1 by 80.7% after 72 h [111].

Although probiotic bacterial strains are more desirable for AFB1 degradation, the use of whole cultures has less potential for large-scale utilization in the industry, so the use of fractions (cells

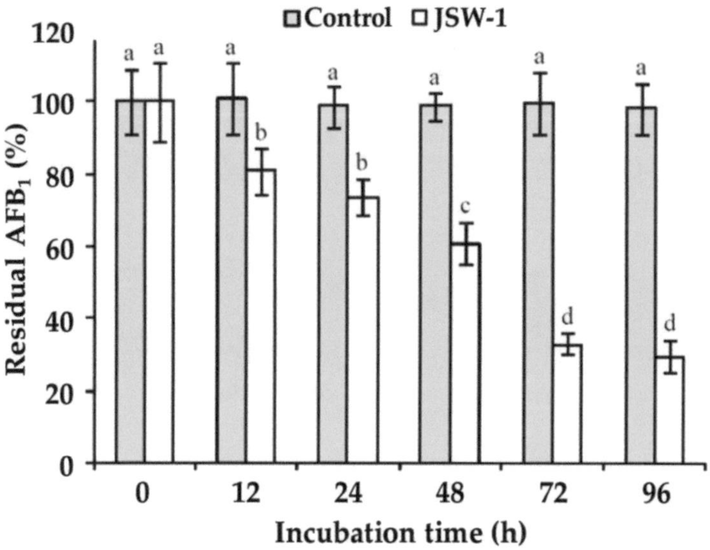

Figure 3. Time course of *in vitro* AFB1 degradation by *B. subtilis* JSW-1 at 30°C for 12, 24, 48, 72, and 96 h in the dark. The initial concentration of AFB1 was 2.5 mg/mL. Values represent the mean ± SD (n = 3). Values with different letters indicate significant differences ($p < 0.05$) among them (modified from [26]).

or lysates) may be convenient, since they are substrate specific, effective, environmentally friendly, and possess better utilization in the food and feed industry [112].

In literature, there are many studies of AFB1 biodegradation carried out in laboratory conditions with many probiotic strains; however, the information in livestock and poultry about the effect of probiotics on AFB1 detoxification is very limited, especially in poultry science. This is important because *in vitro* studies are not always good indicators of the *in vivo* responses, since there are physiological parameters, such as pH, peristaltic movements, and gastric and intestinal secretions affecting their *in vivo* behavior. This can be observed in studies carried out with the genus *Bacillus* spp., of which some strains have been identified as GRAS organisms with probiotic properties in humans and animals as direct fed microbials (DFM). In the *in vitro* study, 3 of 69 *Bacillus* spp. candidates, which were evaluated, showed ability to biodegrade AFB1, based on growth as well as reduction of fluorescence and area of clearance around each colony [70]. However, when the biodegradation potential of these selected *Bacillus* spp. was tested in broiler chickens, no beneficial performance effects were showed. In addition, no significant performance differences were observed when compared with their respective control diets [113]. Therefore, there is still missing research to evaluate the effect of AFB1 degrading probiotics on growth performance, digestibility, immune function, and toxic residues in tissues and excreta in livestock production animals.

The other mechanism that the probiotics have to counteract the toxic effects of AFB1 is through its physical adsorption, which is in fact the most commonly used technique for reducing exposure to AFB1 [114]. It has been demonstrated that AFB1 is absorbed into the enterocytes by passive diffusion so, after its oral ingestion, AFB1 is efficiently absorbed in the intestinal tract, being the duodenum the major site of absorption [115]. If the AFB1 is physically linked to the probiotic microorganism, its bioavailability is decreased, and therefore AFB1 uptake and its access to systemic circulation are also diminished. Adsorption is a physical process, in which the cell wall of microorganism binds the toxin by non-covalent weak bonds and some electrostatic attraction. This interaction appears to occur predominantly with polysaccharides, peptidoglycan, and teichoic or lipoteichoic acids in the cell wall [116–118].

In vitro adsorption of AFB1 by probiotics has been described as a fast and reversible process, which is affected for many factors such as strain, toxin dose, temperature, pH, and microorganism concentration [72, 104, 118–120]. It has also been demonstrated that viability of some probiotic strain does not affect their absorption ability; thus, viable, heat-killed, and acid-killed cells respond in a similar manner [118, 121].

Several studies have been done in optimal laboratory conditions with several strains of probiotic microorganisms tested for their capacity to adsorb AFB1 and have been reported a wide range of genus, species, and strain-specific binding capacities [75, 81, 104, 116, 122–125], being the LABs and yeasts such as *Saccharomyces cerevisiae* those that have demonstrated the greatest ability to remove AFB1 by its adsorption [126]. Such is the case of *Lactobacillus rhamnosus* GG and *Lb. rhamnosus* LC-705, which have demonstrated to be very effective for removing AFB1, being able to remove up to 80% of the toxin instantly [104, 127]. On the other hand, yeasts have been reported to have similar mechanism as LAB in binding to AFB1 as a means of detoxification [68, 126], with studies that have shown that some strains of *S. cerevisiae* can adsorb up to 90% of AFB1 [123, 128].

There is strong evidence in literature that some specific probiotics can adsorb AFB1 *in vitro*, but only limited information is available on adsorption in poultry *in vivo*. These *in vivo* studies are really important since *in vitro* studies have shown that there are relevant physiological conditions that the microorganisms encounter during their passage through the gastrointestinal tract, such as pH, intestinal mucus, and presence of bile, which modify the AFB1 adsorption and the stability of the AFB1-microorganism complex, either positively or negatively [122]. Although not many probiotic strains have been tested *in vivo*, the studies that have been conducted in poultry showed good results, such as in the *in vivo* study using the chicken duodenum loop technique, in which probiotic strain GG of *L. rhamnosus* removed as high as 54% of the added AFB1 and reduced its intestinal adsorption by 73% [73]. In this study, there was a difference in adsorption capacity when these strains were incubated *in vitro*, being the reduction of AFB1 even higher *in vivo* when compared to its adsorption *in vitro*. *Bacillus* probiotics have also been proved to remove or reduce AFB1 adsorption in the gastrointestinal tract at *in vivo* and *in vitro* conditions, showing the positive impact of these bacteria in preventing the harmful effects of aflatoxin in poultry with regard to performance, serum biochemistry, and immune responses [69]. However, when the capacity of *Bacillus* and *Lactobacilli* strains to control the stressful effects caused for AFB1 on chickens was compared, the *Lactobacilli* abilities resulted to be higher. This study shows that these probiotics can control the toxicity of AFB on poultry by improving humoral and cellular immune function, serum biochemical parameters, the process of protein synthesis, and reducing the anti-nutritional effects of AFB1 [65]. In a recent study, the effect of lactic acid bacteria and HSCAS on detoxification of AFB was evaluated in broiler chickens. The results showed that LAB or HSCAS supplementation improved the growth performance, digestibility, and immune function of birds, reducing deleterious effects and tissue residues of AFB1; however, the effect of LAB resulted to be more effective than HSCAS, which indicates a possible mechanism of biodegradation of the toxin by the probiotics [129].

5. Use of polymers to prevent AFB1 toxic effects in poultry

As it was mentioned in Section 1, an important approach to prevent aflatoxicosis in livestock and poultry is the addition of non-nutritional adsorbents in the diet to bind AFB1 in the gastrointestinal tract, reducing its bioavailability, which leads to a reduction of mycotoxin uptake as well as distribution to the blood and the target organs. These adsorbents are large molecular weight compounds that are able to bind the mycotoxin, forming a stable complex adsorbent-mycotoxin, which can pass through the gastrointestinal tract of the animals without dissociating the AFB1, to be eliminated via the feces [22].

The efficacy of adsorption appears to depend on the chemical structure of both the adsorbent, the mycotoxin, and the feed components. The physicochemical properties of the adsorbents such as total charge, charge distribution, size of the pores on the surface, surface area, iodine number, methylene blue index, and pH take on an important function in binding effectively. On the other hand, the properties of the adsorbed mycotoxins, like polarity, solubility, size, shape, charge distribution, and dissociation constants, also play a significant role. It has also been mentioned that the high fiber content of the feed substrate increased the mycotoxin affinity to adsorbent [17, 18].

Even though clay minerals and aluminosilicate materials have been tested and recognized for their ability to bind AFB1 successfully [130, 131], the main risk of using them in animal feed is that they can also adsorb some feed vitamins and minerals, decreasing their utilization by animals [132, 133]. Another risk is that clays can release toxic components or elements bound to them, as heavy metals or dioxins, which can be released in the intestine of animals and accumulated in animal organs [134, 135].

Facing the problems of the use of clay and aluminosilicate adsorbents, other types of binders have been investigated in the search for new adsorbent materials such as organic binders or biopolymers and synthetic polymers [17, 112]. Both kind of polymers are large molecules that are composed of many monomers, whose large molecular mass relative to a small molecule produces unique physical properties playing important roles in our society [24]. Just a few synthetic polymers have been evaluated and demonstrated to bind mycotoxins *in vitro* and *in vivo*, such as cholestyramine, divinylbenzene-styrene, polyvinylpyrrolidone (PVP), and its modification polyvinylpolypyrrolidone (PVPP) [7, 17, 18, 112]; nevertheless, from these polymers, only PVP and PVPP have been tested against AFB1 in poultry. *In vitro* studies indicate that PVPP can bind up to 50 mg/kg of AFB1 from feed. On the other hand, *in vivo* studies carried out in broiler chickens demonstrated that PVPP could have ameliorated some serum biochemical and hematological parameters, it might have meliorated the detrimental effects of AFB1 on the immune system, and that the pathological changes were markedly inhibited by the administration of PVPP in the diet [136–139]. However, the cost of those polymers would be a limiting factor for practical applications.

Biopolymers are generally complex indigestible carbohydrates, non-toxic, biocompatible, and biodegradable, such as cellulose, cellulose, lignin, hemicellulose, glucomannans, peptidoglycans, and chitosan. They have been widely used as a promising biosorbents for the removal of various heavy metal ions and dyes [140], but recently cellulosic polymers and chitosan have been demonstrated to have ability to adsorb AFB1 [24, 141]. According to the *in vitro* results, both cellulosic polymers and chitosan were able to bind other important mycotoxins for poultry industry besides AFB1, which is a clear advantage over inorganic adsorbents since they are very effective in preventing aflatoxicosis, but their efficacy against mycotoxins such as zearalenone, ochratoxin, and trichothecenes is limited [17]. These biopolymers also pose multilayer porous structure filled with openings and channels that provide huge volume per sorbent surface unit, which is favorable in the adsorption process. Concerning to chitosan, different molecular weights, deacetylation degree, and cross-linked degree have to be tested for their AFB1 adsorption properties, because these characteristics might show different adsorptive capacity against this mycotoxin [24].

The results on the efficacy of polymers in sequestering mycotoxins are highly promising, although this field is still in its infancy and further research is needed. Furthermore, *in vivo* studies are needed to confirm the effectiveness of these materials against AFB1 toxic effects, since results in the past have indicated that there is great variability in the efficacy of adsorbing materials *in vivo*, even though the compounds may show potential adsorption capacity of the mycotoxin *in vitro* [22].

Author details

Bruno Solis-Cruz[1], Daniel Hernandez-Patlan[1], Billy M. Hargis[2] and Guillermo Tellez[2]*

*Address all correspondence to: gtellez@uark.edu

1 National Autonomous University of Mexico-Superior Studies Faculty at Cuautitlan (UNAM-FESC), Multidisciplinary Research Unit L5 (Pharmaceutical Development Testing Laboratory), Cuautitlan Izcalli, Mexico

2 Department of Poultry Science, University of Arkansas, Fayetteville, AR, USA

References

[1] Hussein HS, Brasel JM. Toxicity, metabolism, and impact of mycotoxins on humans and animals. Toxicology. 2001;**167**(2):101-134

[2] Adebo O, Njobeh P, Gbashi S, Nwinyi O, Mavumengwana V. Review on microbial degradation of aflatoxins. Critical Reviews in Food Science and Nutrition. 2017;**57**(15): 3208-3217

[3] Kabak B, Dobson ADW, Var I. Strategies to prevent mycotoxin contamination of food and animal feed: A review. Critical Reviews in Food Science and Nutrition. 2006;**46**(8): 593-619

[4] Bondy GS, Pestka JJ. Immunomodulation by fungal toxins. Journal of Toxicology and Environmental Health Part B: Critical Reviews. 2000;**3**(2):109-143

[5] Coulombe RA Jr. Biological action of mycotoxins. Journal of Dairy Science. 1993;**76**(3): 880-891

[6] Rawal S, Kim JE, Coulombe R. Aflatoxin B1 in poultry: Toxicology, metabolism and prevention. Research in Veterinary Science. 2010;**89**(3):325-331

[7] Jouany JP. Methods for preventing, decontaminating and minimizing the toxicity of mycotoxins in feeds. Animal Feed Science and Technology. 2007;**137**(3–4):342-362

[8] Commission CA, Commission CA, et al. Code of practice for the prevention and reduction of mycotoxin contamination of cereals, including annexes on ochratoxin a, zearalenone, fumonisins and trichothecenes. CAC/RCP. 2003;51-2003

[9] McKenzie KS, Sarr AB, Mayura K, Bailey RH, Miller DR, Rogers TD, et al. Oxidative degradation and detoxification of mycotoxins using a novel source of ozone. Food and Chemical Toxicology. 1997;**35**(8):807-820

[10] Goldblatt L, Dollear F. Review of prevention, elimination, and detoxification of aflatoxins. Pure and Applied Chemistry. 1977;**49**(11):1759-1764

[11] Ghosh M, Chhabra A, Atreja P, Chopra R. Effect of treating with propionic acid, sodium bisulfite and sodium hydroxide on the biosynthesis of aflatoxin on groundnut cake. Animal Feed Science and Technology. 1996;**60**(1):43-49

[12] Aziz NH, El-Zeany SA, LAA M. Influence of gamma-irradiation and maize lipids on the production of aflatoxin B1 by *Aspergillus flavus*. Die Nahrung. 2002;**46**(5):327-331

[13] Samarajeewa U, Sen A, Cohen M, Wei C. Detoxification of aflatoxins in foods and feeds by physical and chemical methods. Journal of Food Protection. International Association for Food Protection. 1990;**53**(6):489-501

[14] Pankaj S, Shi H, Keener KM. A review of novel physical and chemical decontamination technologies for aflatoxin in food. Trends in Food Science & Technology. 2017;**71**:73-83

[15] Kubena L, Harvey R, Bailey R, Buckley S, Rottinghaus G. Effects of a hydrated sodium calcium aluminosilicate (T-bind) on mycotoxicosis in young broiler chickens. Poultry Science. 1998;**77**(10):1502-1509

[16] Kong C, Shin SY, Kim BG. Evaluation of mycotoxin sequestering agents for aflatoxin and deoxynivalenol: An in vitro approach. SpringerPlus. 2014;**3**(1):346

[17] Huwig A, Freimund S, Käppeli O, Dutler H. Mycotoxin detoxification of animal feed by different adsorbents. Toxicology Letters. 2001;**122**(2):179-188

[18] Avantaggiato G, Solfrizzo M, Visconti A. Recent advances on the use of adsorbent materials for detoxification of *Fusarium mycotoxins*. Food Additives and Contaminants. 2005;**22**(4):379-388

[19] Dixon J, Kannewischer I, Arvide MT, Velazquez AB. Aflatoxin sequestration in animal feeds by quality-labeled smectite clays: An introductory plan. Applied Clay Science. 2008;**40**(1–4):201-208

[20] Jaynes W, Zartman R, Hudnall W. Aflatoxin B1 adsorption by clays from water and corn meal. Applied Clay Science. 2007;**36**(1–3):197-205

[21] Papaioannou D, Katsoulos P, Panousis N, Karatzias H. The role of natural and synthetic zeolites as feed additives on the prevention and/or the treatment of certain farm animal diseases: A review. Microporous and Mesoporous Materials. 2005;**84**(1–3):161-170

[22] Boudergue C, Burel C, Dragacci S, Favrot M-C, Fremy J-M, Massimi C, et al. Review of mycotoxin-detoxifying agents used as feed additives: Mode of action, efficacy and feed/food safety. EFSA Supporting Publications. 2009;**6**(9):1-192

[23] Kolosova A, Stroka J. Evaluation of the effect of mycotoxin binders in animal feed on the analytical performance of standardised methods for the determination of mycotoxins in feed. Food Additives & Contaminants: Part A. 2012;**29**(12):1959-1971

[24] Solis-Cruz B, Hernández-Patlán D, Beyssac E, Latorre JD, Hernandez-Velasco X, Merino-Guzman R, et al. Evaluation of chitosan and cellulosic polymers as binding adsorbent materials to prevent aflatoxin B1, fumonisin B1, ochratoxin, trichothecene, deoxynivalenol, and zearalenone mycotoxicoses through an in vitro gastrointestinal model for poultry. Polymers. 2017;**9**(10):529

[25] Zuo R, Chang J, Yin Q, Wang P, Yang Y, Wang X, et al. Effect of the combined probiotics with aflatoxin B1-degrading enzyme on aflatoxin detoxification, broiler production performance and hepatic enzyme gene expression. Food and Chemical Toxicology. 2013;**59**:470-475

[26] Xia X, Zhang Y, Li M, Garba B, Zhang Q, Wang Y, et al. Isolation and characterization of a *Bacillus subtilis* strain with aflatoxin B1 biodegradation capability. Food Control. 2017;**75**:92-98

[27] Slizewska K, Smulikowska S. Detoxification of aflatoxin B1 and change in microflora pattern by probiotic in vitro fermentation of broiler feed. Journal of Animal and Feed Sciences. 2011;**20**:300-309

[28] Rawal S, Bauer MM, Mendoza KM, El-Nezami H, Hall JR, Kim JE, et al. Aflatoxicosis chemoprevention by probiotic Lactobacillus and lack of effect on the major histocompatibility complex. Research in veterinary science. 2014;**97**(2):274-281

[29] Halasz A, Lásztity R, Abonyi T, Bata Á. Decontamination of mycotoxin-containing food and feed by biodegradation. Food Reviews International. 2009;**25**(4):284-298

[30] Aliabadi MA, Alikhani FE, Mohammadi M, Darsanaki RK. Biological control of aflatoxins. European Journal of Experimental Biology. 2013;**3**(2):162-166

[31] Vinderola G, Ritieni A. Role of probiotics against mycotoxins and their deleterious effects. Journal of Food Research. 2014;**4**(1):10

[32] Tipu M, Saleem U, Rehman T, Aslam M, Muhammad K, Hussain K, et al. Protective role of *Lactobacillus acidophilus* against aflatoxin B1 induced immunosuppression. JAPS. Journal of Animal and Plant Sciences. 2015;**25**(6):1566-1571

[33] Kurhan S, Çakir I. DNA-bioprotective effects of lactic acid bacteria against aflatoxin B1. Current Research in Nutrition and Food Science Journal. 2016;**4**(Special Issue Nutrition in Conference October 2016):87-91

[34] Coulombe RA, Guarisco JA, Klein PJ, Hall JO. Chemoprevention of aflatoxicosis in poultry by dietary butylated hydroxytoluene. Animal Feed Science and Technology. 2005;**121**(1–2):217-225

[35] Dalvi R. An overview of aflatoxicosis of poultry: Its characteristics, prevention and reduction. Veterinary Research Communications. 1986;**10**(1):429-443

[36] Greco MV, Franchi ML, Rico Golba SL, Pardo AG, Pose GN. Mycotoxins and mycotoxigenic fungi in poultry feed for food-producing animals. The Scientific World Journal. 2014;**2014**:1-9

[37] Huff W, Kubena L, Harvey R, Corrier D, Mollenhauer H. Progression of aflatoxicosis in broiler chickens. Poultry Science. 1986;**65**(10):1891-1899

[38] Smith J, Hamilton P. Aflatoxicosis in the broiler chicken. Poultry science. 1970;**49**(1):207-215

[39] Mottet A, Tempio G. Global poultry production: Current state and future outlook and challenges. World's Poultry Science Journal. 2017;**73**(2):245-256

[40] Muller R, Carlson C, Semeniuk G, Harshfield G. The response of chicks, ducklings, goslings, pheasants and poults to graded levels of aflatoxins. Poultry Science. 1970; **49**(5):1346-1350

[41] Mishra HN, Das C. A review on biological control and metabolism of aflatoxin. Critical Reviews in Food Science and Nutrition. 2003;**43**(3):245-264

[42] Smela ME, Currier SS, Bailey EA, Essigmann JM. The chemistry and biology of aflatoxin B(1): From mutational spectrometry to carcinogenesis. Carcinogenesis. 2001;**22**(4):535-545

[43] Bbosa GS, Kitya D, Lubega A, Ogwal-Okeng J, Anokbonggo WW, Kyegombe DB. Review of the biological and health effects of aflatoxins on body organs and body systems. Aflatoxins-Recent Advances and Future Prospects. 2013;**12**:239-265

[44] McKean C, Tang L, Tang M, Billam M, Wang Z, Theodorakis CW, et al. Comparative acute and combinative toxicity of aflatoxin B1 and fumonisin B1 in animals and human cells. Food and Chemical Toxicology. 2006;**44**(6):868-876

[45] Lozano M, Diaz G. Microsomal and cytosolic biotransformation of aflatoxin B1 in four poultry species. British Poultry Science. 2006;**47**(6):734-41

[46] Gregorio MCD, Bordin K, Souto PCM de C, Corassin CH, CAF O. Comparative biotransformation of aflatoxin B1 in swine, domestic fowls, and humans. Toxin Reviews. 2015; **34**(3):142-150

[47] Diaz GJ, Murcia HW. Biotransformation of aflatoxin B1 and its relationship with the differential toxicological response to aflatoxin in commercial poultry species. Aflatoxins-Biochemistry and Molecular Biology. 2011;**1**:3-20

[48] Jones F, Hagler W, Hamilton P. Association of low levels of aflatoxin in feed with productivity losses in commercial broiler operations. Poultry Science. 1982;**61**(5):861-868

[49] Khlangwiset P, Shephard GS, Wu F. Aflatoxins and growth impairment: A review. Critical Reviews in Toxicology. 2011;**41**(9):740-755

[50] Moorthy A, Mahendar M, Rao P. Hepatopathology in experimental aflatoxicosis in chickens. Indian Journal of Animal Sciences (India). 1985;**55**:629-632

[51] Hussain Z, Khan MZ, Hassan Z. Production of aflatoxins from *Aspergillus flavus* and acute aflatoxicosis in young broiler chicks. Pakistan Journal of Agricultural Sciences. 2008;**45**(1):95-102

[52] Quezada T, Cuellar H, Jaramillo-Juarez F, Valdivia A, Reyes J. Effects of aflatoxin B1 on the liver and kidney of broiler chickens during development. Comparative Biochemistry and Physiology Part C: Pharmacology, Toxicology and Endocrinology. 2000;**125**(3):265-272

[53] Qureshi M, Brake J, Hamilton P, Hagler W Jr, Nesheim S. Dietary exposure of broiler breeders to aflatoxin results in immune dysfunction in progeny chicks. Poultry Science. 1998;**77**(6):812-819

[54] Ghosh R, Chauhan H, Jha G. Suppression of cell-mediated immunity by purified aflatoxin B1 in broiler chicks. Veterinary Immunology and Immunopathology. 1991;**28**(2): 165-172

[55] Azzam A, Gabal M. Interaction of aflatoxin in the feed and immunization against selected infectious diseases. I. Infectious bursal disease. Avian Pathology. 1997;**26**(2):317-325

[56] Gabal M, Azzam A. Interaction of aflatoxin in the feed and immunization against selected infectious diseases in poultry. II. Effect on one-day-old layer chicks simultaneously vaccinated against Newcastle disease, infectious bronchitis and infectious bursal disease. Avian Pathology. 1998;**27**(3):290-295

[57] Bryden WL. Mycotoxin contamination of the feed supply chain: Implications for animal productivity and feed security. Animal Feed Science and Technology. 2012;**173**(1–2):134-158

[58] Grenier B, Loureiro-Bracarense A-P, Leslie JF, Oswald IP. Physical and chemical methods for mycotoxin decontamination in maize. Mycotoxin Reduct Grain Chains. 2014;**9**:116-129

[59] Verheecke C, Liboz T, Mathieu F. Microbial degradation of aflatoxin B1: Current status and future advances. International Journal of Food Microbiology. 2016;**237**:1-9

[60] Young JC, Zhou T, Yu H, Zhu H, Gong J. Degradation of trichothecene mycotoxins by chicken intestinal microbes. Food and Chemical Toxicology. 2007;**45**(1):136-143

[61] Ciegler A, Lillehoj E, Peterson R, Hall H. Microbial detoxification of aflatoxin. Applied Microbiology. 1966;**14**(6):934-939

[62] Magan N, Olsen M. Mycotoxins in Food: Detection and Control. Cambridge, UK: Woodhead Publishing Ltd; 2004

[63] Poloni V, Dogi C, Pereyra CM, Fernández Juri MG, Köhler P, Rosa CA, et al. Potentiation of the effect of a commercial animal feed additive mixed with different probiotic yeast strains on the adsorption of aflatoxin B1. Food Additives & Contaminants: Part A. 2015; **32**(6):970-976

[64] Karabulut S, Paytakov G, Leszczynski J. Reduction of aflatoxin B1 to aflatoxicol: A comprehensive DFT study provides clues to its toxicity. Journal of the Science of Food and Agriculture. 2014;**94**(15):3134-3140

[65] Barati M, Chamani M, Mousavi SN, Hoseini SA, Taj Abadi Ebrahimi M. Effects of biological and mineral compounds in aflatoxin-contaminated diets on blood parameters and immune response of broiler chickens. Journal of Applied Animal Research. 2018; **46**(1):707-713

[66] Gacem MA, El Hadj-Khelil AO. Toxicology, biosynthesis, bio-control of aflatoxin and new methods of detection. Asian Pacific Journal of Tropical Biomedicine. 2016;**6**(9):808-814

[67] Ji C, Fan Y, Zhao L. Review on biological degradation of mycotoxins. Animal Nutrition. 2016;**2**(3):127-133

[68] Wu Q, Jezkova A, Yuan Z, Pavlikova L, Dohnal V, Kuca K. Biological degradation of aflatoxins. Drug Metabolism Reviews. 2009;**41**(1):1-7

[69] Bagherzadeh KF, Karimi TM, Allameh A, Shariatmadari F. A novel aflatoxin-binding Bacillus probiotic: Performance, serum biochemistry, and immunological parameters in Japanese quail. Poultry Science. 2012;**91**(8):1846

[70] Galarza-Seeber R, Latorre JD, Hernandez-Velasco X, Wolfenden AD, Bielke LR, Menconi A, et al. Isolation, screening and identification of Bacillus spp. as direct-fed microbial candidates for aflatoxin B1 biodegradation. Asian Pacific. Journal of Tropical Biomedicine. 2015;**5**(9):702-706

[71] Gao X, Ma Q, Zhao L, Lei Y, Shan Y, Ji C. Isolation of *Bacillus subtilis*: Screening for aflatoxins B1, M1, and G1 detoxification. European Food Research and Technology. 2011; **232**(6):957

[72] Bueno DJ, Casale CH, Pizzolitto RP, Salvano MA, Oliver G. Physical adsorption of aflatoxin B1 by lactic acid bacteria and *Saccharomyces cerevisiae*: A theoretical model. Journal of Food Protection. International Association for Food Protection. 2007;**70**(9):2148-2154

[73] El-Nezami H, Mykkänen H, Kankaanpää P, Salminen S, Ahokas J. Ability of Lactobacillus and Propionibacterium strains to remove aflatoxin B, from the chicken duodenum. Journal of Food Protection. 2000;**63**(4):549

[74] Hamidi A, Mirnejad R, Yahaghi E, Behnod V, Mirhosseini A, Amani S, et al. The aflatoxin B1 isolating potential of two lactic acid bacteria. Asian Pacific Journal of Tropical Biomedicine. 2013;**3**(9):732-736

[75] Haskard CA, El-Nezami HS, Kankaanpää PE, Salminen S, Ahokas JT. Surface binding of aflatoxin B1 by lactic acid bacteria. Applied and Environmental Microbiology. 2001;**67**(7): 3086-3091

[76] Nada S, Amra H, Deabes M, Omara E. *Saccharomyces cerevisiae* and probiotic bacteria potentially inhibit aflatoxins production in vitro and in vivo studies. International Journal of Toxicology. 2010;**8**(1):32

[77] Fijan S. Microorganisms with claimed probiotic properties: An overview of recent literature. International Journal of Environmental Research and Public Health. 2014;**11**(5):4745-4767

[78] Patterson J, Burkholder K. Application of prebiotics and probiotics in poultry production. Poultry Science. 2003;**82**(4):627-631

[79] Park YH, Hamidon F, Rajangan C, Soh KP, Gan CY, Lim TS, et al. Application of probiotics for the production of safe and high-quality poultry meat. Korean Journal for Food Science of Animal Resources. 2016;**36**(5):567

[80] Kabir S. The role of probiotics in the poultry industry. International Journal of Molecular Sciences. 2009;**10**(8):3531-3546

[81] Peltonen KD, El-Nezami HS, Salminen SJ, Ahokas JT. Binding of aflatoxin B1 by probiotic bacteria. Journal of the Science of Food and Agriculture. 2000;**80**(13):1942-1945

[82] Gourama H, Bullerman LB. Inhibition of growth and aflatoxin production of *Aspergillus flavus* by Lactobacillus species. Journal of Food Protection. International Association for Food Protection. 1995;**58**(11):1249-1256

[83] Gerbaldo GA, Barberis C, Pascual L, Dalcero A, Barberis L. Antifungal activity of two Lactobacillus strains with potential probiotic properties. FEMS Microbiology Letters. 2012;**332**(1):27-33

[84] Bueno DJ, Silva JO, Oliver G, Gonzalez SN. *Lactobacillus casei* CRL 431 and *Lactobacillus rhamnosus* CRL 1224 as biological controls for *Aspergillus flavus* strains. Journal of Food Protection. 2006;**69**(10):2544-2548

[85] Onilude A, Fagade O, Bello M, Fadahunsi I. Inhibition of aflatoxin-producing aspergilli by lactic acid bacteria isolates from indigenously fermented cereal gruels. African Journal of Biotechnology. 2005;**4**(12):1404-1408

[86] Reddy K, Raghavender C, Reddy B, Salleh B. Biological control of *Aspergillus flavus* growth and subsequent aflatoxin B 1 production in sorghum grains. African Journal of Biotechnology. 2010;**9**(27):4247-4250

[87] Prathivadi Bayankaram P, Sellamuthu PS. Antifungal and anti-aflatoxigenic effect of probiotics against *Aspergillus flavus* and *Aspergillus parasiticus*. Toxin Reviews. 2016;**35** (1–2):10-15

[88] Cole RJ, Cotty PJ. Biocontrol of aflatoxin production by using biocompetitive agents. In: A Perspective on Aflatoxin in Field Crops and Animal Food Products in the United States: A Symposium. 1990. pp. 62-66

[89] Lee L, Dunn J, DeLucca A, Ciegler A. Role of lactone ring of aflatoxin B 1 in toxicity and mutagenicity. Experientia. 1981;**37**(1):16-17

[90] Samuel SM, Aiko V, Panda P, Mehta A. Aflatoxin B-1 occurrence, biosynthesis and its degradation. Journal of Pure and Applied Microbiology. 2013;**7**(2):965-971

[91] Mokoena M, Chelule P, Gqaleni N. The toxicity and decreased concentration of aflatoxin B1 in natural lactic acid fermented maize meal. Journal of Applied Microbiology. 2006; **100**(4):773-777

[92] Cao H, Liu D, Mo X, Xie C, Yao D. A fungal enzyme with the ability of aflatoxin B1 conversion: Purification and ESI-MS/MS identification. Microbiological Research. 2011; **166**(6):475-483

[93] Mao J, He B, Zhang L, Li P, Zhang Q, Ding X, et al. A structure identification and toxicity assessment of the degradation products of aflatoxin B1 in peanut oil under UV irradiation. Toxins. 2016;**8**(11):332

[94] Ghazvini RD, Kouhsari E, Zibafar E, Hashemi SJ, Amini A, Niknejad F. Antifungal activity and aflatoxin degradation of *Bifidobacterium bifidum* and *Lactobacillus fermentum* against toxigenic *Aspergillus parasiticus*. The Open Microbiology Journal. 2016;**10**:197

[95] Farzaneh M, Shi Z-Q, Ghassempour A, Sedaghat N, Ahmadzadeh M, Mirabolfathy M, et al. Aflatoxin B1 degradation by *Bacillus subtilis* UTBSP1 isolated from pistachio nuts of Iran. Food Control. 2012;**23**(1):100-106

[96] Taylor MC, Jackson CJ, Tattersall DB, French N, Peat TS, Newman J, et al. Identification and characterization of two families of F420H2-dependent reductases from Mycobacteria that catalyse aflatoxin degradation. Molecular Microbiology. 2010;**78**(3): 561-575

[97] Teniola O, Addo P, Brost I, Färber P, Jany K-D, Alberts J, et al. Degradation of aflatoxin B1 by cell-free extracts of *Rhodococcus erythropolis* and *Mycobacterium fluoranthenivorans* sp. nov. DSM44556T. International Journal of Food Microbiology. 2005;**105**(2):111-117

[98] Adebo OA, Njobeh PB, Mavumengwana V. Degradation and detoxification of AFB1 by *Staphylococcus warneri*, *Sporosarcina* sp. and *Lysinibacillus fusiformis*. Food Control. 2016; **68**:92-96

[99] Adebo OA, Njobeh PB, Sidu S, Tlou MG, Mavumengwana V. Aflatoxin B1 degradation by liquid cultures and lysates of three bacterial strains. International Journal of Food Microbiology. 2016;**233**:11-19

[100] Mann R, Rehm H-J. Degradation products from aflatoxin B1 by *Corynebacterium rubrum, Aspergillus niger, Trichoderma viride* and *Mucor ambiguus*. European Journal of applied Microbiology and Biotechnology. 1976;**2**(4):297-306

[101] Tsubouchi H, Yamamoto K, Hisada K, Sakabe Y. Degradation of aflatoxins by *Aspergillus niger* and aflatoxin non-producing *Aspergillus flavus*. Journal of the Food Hygienic Society of Japan (Japan). 1983;**24**(2):113-119

[102] Eshelli M, Harvey L, Edrada-Ebel R, McNeil B. Metabolomics of the bio-degradation process of aflatoxin B1 by actinomycetes at an initial pH of 6.0. Toxins. 2015;**7**(2):439-456

[103] Huynh V, Gerdes R, Lloyd A. Synthesis and degradation of aflatoxins by *Aspergillus parasiticus*. II. Comparative toxicity and mutagenicity of aflatoxin B1 and it autolytic breakdown products. Australian Journal of Biological Sciences. 1984;**37**(3):123-130

[104] El-Nezami H, Kankaanpaa P, Salminen S, Ahokas J. Ability of dairy strains of lactic acid bacteria to bind a common food carcinogen, aflatoxin B1. Food and Chemical Toxicology. 1998;**36**(4):321-326

[105] Oatley JT, Rarick MD, Ji GE, Linz JE. Binding of aflatoxin B1 to bifidobacteria in vitro. Journal of Food Protection. 2000;**63**(8):1133-1136

[106] Peltonen K, El-Nezami H, Haskard C, Ahokas J, Salminen S. Aflatoxin B1 binding by dairy strains of lactic acid bacteria and bifidobacteria. Journal of Dairy Science. 2001; **84**(10):2152-2156

[107] Guan S, Ji C, Zhou T, Li J, Ma Q, Niu T. Aflatoxin B1 degradation by *Stenotrophomonas maltophilia* and other microbes selected using coumarin medium, International Journal of Molecular Sciences. 2008;**9**(8):1489-1503

[108] Hormisch D, Brost I, Kohring G-W, Giffhorn F, Kroppenstedt R, Stackebradt E, et al. *Mycobacterium fluoranthenivorans* sp. nov., a fluoranthene and aflatoxin B1 degrading bacterium from contaminated soil of a former coal gas plant. Systematic and Applied Microbiology. 2004;**27**(6):653-660

[109] Smiley R, Draughon F. Preliminary evidence that degradation of aflatoxin B1 by *Flavobacterium aurantiacum* is enzymatic. Journal of Food Protection. 2000;**63**(3):415-418

[110] Tejada-Castaneda Z, Avila-Gonzalez E, Casaubon-Huguenin M, Cervantes-Olivares R, Vásquez-Peláez C, Hernandez-Baumgarten E, et al. Biodetoxification of aflatoxin-contaminated chick feed. Poultry Science. 2008;**87**(8):1569-1576

[111] Guan S, Zhao L, Ma Q, Zhou T, Wang N, Hu X, et al. In vitro efficacy of *Myxococcus fulvus* ANSM068 to biotransform aflatoxin B1. International Journal of Molecular Sciences. 2010;**11**(10):4063-4079

[112] Kolosova A, Stroka J. Substances for reduction of the contamination of feed by mycotoxins: A review. World Mycotoxin Journal. 2011;**4**(3):225-256

[113] Galarza-Seeber R, Latorre J, Wolfenden A, Hernandez-Velasco X, Merino-Guzman R, Ledoux D, et al. Evaluation of Bacillus spp. as direct fed microbial (DFM) candidates for

aflatoxin B1 biodegradation in broiler chickens. International Journal of Probiotics & Prebiotics. 2016;**11**(1):29

[114] Hathout AS, Aly SE. Biological detoxification of mycotoxins: A review. Annals of Microbiology. 2014;**64**(3):905-919

[115] Hsieh DP, Wong JJ. Pharmacokinetics and excretion of aflatoxins. In: The Toxicology of Aflatoxins: Human Health, Veterinary, and Agricultural Significance. San Diego, CA: Academic Press. pp. 73-88

[116] Damayanti E, Istiqomah L, Saragih J, Purwoko T, et al. Characterization of lactic acid bacteria as poultry probiotic candidates with aflatoxin B1 binding activities. IOP Conference Series: Earth and Environmental Science. 2017. p. 012030

[117] Gratz S, Mykkänen H, El-Nezami H. Aflatoxin B1 binding by a mixture of Lactobacillus and Propionibacterium: In vitro versus ex vivo. Journal of Food Protection. 2005;**68**(11): 2470-2474

[118] Haskard C, Binnion C, Ahokas J. Factors affecting the sequestration of aflatoxin by *Lactobacillus rhamnosus* strain GG. Chemico-biological Interactions. 2000;**128**(1):39-49

[119] Kankaanpää P, Tuomola E, El-Nezami H, Ahokas J, Salminen S, et al. Binding of aflatoxin B1 alters the adhesion properties of *Lactobacillus rhamnosus* strain GG in a Caco-2 model. Journal of Food Protection. 2000;**63**(3):412-414

[120] El Khoury A, Atoui A, Yaghi J. Analysis of aflatoxin M1 in milk and yogurt and AFM1 reduction by lactic acid bacteria used in Lebanese industry. Food Control. 2011;**22**(10): 1695-1699

[121] El-Nezami H, Kankaanpää P, Salminen S, Ahokas J. Physicochemical alterations enhance the ability of dairy strains of lactic acid bacteria to remove aflatoxin from contaminated media. Journal of Food Protection. 1998;**61**(4):466-468

[122] Hernandez-Mendoza A, Garcia H, Steele J. Screening of *Lactobacillus casei* strains for their ability to bind aflatoxin B1. Food and Chemical Toxicology. 2009;**47**(6):1064-1068

[123] Gonçalves BL, Rosim RE, de Oliveira CAF, Corassin CH. The in vitro ability of different *Saccharomyces cerevisiae*-based products to bind aflatoxin B1. Food Control. 2015;**47**:298-300

[124] Fazeli MR, Hajimohammadali M, Moshkani A, Samadi N, Jamalifar H, Khoshayand MR, et al. Aflatoxin B1 binding capacity of autochthonous strains of lactic acid bacteria. Journal of Food Protection. 2009;**72**(1):189-192

[125] Bagherzadeh Kasmani F, Torshizi K, Allameh A, Shariatmadari F. Aflatoxin detoxification potential of lactic acid bacteria isolated from Iranian poultry. Iranian Journal of Veterinary Research. 2012;**13**(2):152-155

[126] Shetty PH, Jespersen L. *Saccharomyces cerevisiae* and lactic acid bacteria as potential mycotoxin decontaminating agents. Trends in Food Science and Technology. 2006;**17**(2):48-55

[127] Turbic A, Ahokas J, Haskard C. Selective in vitro binding of dietary mutagens, individually or in combination, by lactic acid bacteria. Food Additives and Contaminants. 2002; **19**(2):144-152

[128] Shetty PH, Hald B, Jespersen L. Surface binding of aflatoxin B 1 by *Saccharomyces cerevisiae* strains with potential decontaminating abilities in indigenous fermented foods. International Journal of Food Microbiology. 2007;**113**(1):41-46

[129] Liu N, Wang J, Deng Q, Gu K, Wang J. Detoxification of aflatoxin B1 by lactic acid bacteria and hydrated sodium calcium aluminosilicate in broiler chickens. Livestock Science. 2018;**208**:28-32

[130] Pasha T, Farooq M, Khattak F, Jabbar M, Khan A. Effectiveness of sodium bentonite and two commercial products as aflatoxin absorbents in diets for broiler chickens. Animal Feed Science and Technology. 2007;**132**(1–2):103-110

[131] Phillips TD, Kubena LF, Harvey RB, Taylor DR, Heidelbaugh ND. Hydrated sodium calcium aluminosilicate: A high affinity sorbent for aflatoxin. Poultry Science. 1988;**67**(2): 243-247

[132] Chung T, Ekdman JR, Baker D. Hydrated sodium calcium aluminosilicate: Effects on zinc, manganese, vitamin A, and riboflavin utilization. Poultry Science. 1990;**69**(8):1364-1370

[133] Moshtaghian J, Parsons C, Leeper R, Harrison P, Koelkebeck K. Effect of sodium aluminosilicate on phosphorus utilization by chicks and laying hens. Poultry Science. 1991; **70**(4):955-962

[134] Abad E, Llerena JJ, Sauló J, Caixach J, Rivera J. Comprehensive study on dioxin contents in binder and anti-caking agent feed additives. Chemosphere. 2002;**46**(9–10):1417-1421

[135] Trckova M, Matlova L, Dvorska L, et al. Kaolin, bentonite, and zeolites as feed supplements for animals: Health advantages and risks. A review. Veterinarni Medicina-UZPI (Czech Republic). 2004;**49**:389-399

[136] Celik I, Oğuz H, Demet O, Dönmez HH, Boydak M, Sur E. Efficacy of polyvinylpolypyrrolidone in reducing the immunotoxicity of aflatoxin in growing broilers. British Poultry Science. 2000;**41**(4):430-439

[137] Kececi T, Oguz H, Kurtoglu V, Demet O. Effects of polyvinylpolypyrrolidone, synthetic zeolite and bentonite on serum biochemical and haematological characters of broiler chickens during aflatoxicosis. British Poultry Science. 1998;**39**(3):452-458

[138] Kiran M, Demet Ö, Ortatath M, Oğuz H. The preventive effect of polyvinylpolypyrrolidone on aflatoxicosis in broilers. Avian Pathology. 1998;**27**(3):250-255

[139] Thalib A. Detoxification of aflatoxin in feed with a binder of polyvinylpolypyrrolidone. Jurnal Ilmiah Penelitian Ternak Klepu (Indonesia). 1995;**1**:43-48

[140] Hokkanen S, Bhatnagar A, Sillanpää M. A review on modification methods to cellulose-based adsorbents to improve adsorption capacity. Water research. 2016;**91**:156-173

[141] Zhao Z, Liu N, Yang L, Wang J, Song S, Nie D, et al. Cross-linked chitosan polymers as generic adsorbents for simultaneous adsorption of multiple mycotoxins. Food Control. 2015;**57**:362-369